AROMATHERAPY & MASSAGE

AROMATHERAPY & MASSAGE

ACHIEVING HEALTH AND WELL-BEING THE NATURAL WAY, WITH SIMPLE MASSAGE TECHNIQUES AND AROMATIC TREATMENTS

Sarah Porter & Joanne Rippin

LORENZ BOOKS

First published in 1999 by Lorenz Books

Lorenz Books is an imprint of
Anness Publishing Limited
Hermes House
88–89 Blackfriars Road
London SE1 8HA

This edition distributed in Canada by Raincoast Books,
8680 Cambie Street, Vancouver,
British Columbia V6P 6M9

ISBN 0 7548 0114 4

A CIP catalogue record for this book is available from the British Library

Publisher: Joanna Lorenz
Project Editor: Sarah Duffin
Editor: Beverley Jollands
Aromatherapy Consultant: Anita Glover
Designers: Lilian Lindblom and Bobbie Colgate Stone

Previously published in two separate volumes, *Aromatherapy* and *Massage*

ACKNOWLEDGEMENTS
The publishers would especially like to thank Nitya Lacroix, Carole McGilvery, Jimi Reed and
Sharon Seager who contributed the majority of the text in this book; also Andi Clevely,
Mark Evans, Tessa Evelegh, Gilly Love, Alison Mackonochie, Sally Norton,
Katherine Richmond and Kate Shapland who supplied additional material.
The majority of photographs in the book were taken by Sue Atkinson and Alistair Hughes.
Other photographs were taken by Simon Bottomley, Nick Cole, John Freeman,
Michelle Garrett, Don Last and Debbie Patterson

PICTURE CREDITS
Visual Arts Library: pp 99, 100 and 101

PUBLISHER'S NOTE
The reader should not regard the recommendations, ideas and techniques expressed and
described in this book as substitutes for the advice of a qualified practitioner or other
qualified professional. Any use to which recommendations, ideas and techniques are put is at
the reader's sole discretion.

Printed and bound in Hong Kong/China

1 3 5 7 9 10 8 6 4 2

CONTENTS

$\mathcal{I}$NTRODUCTION

For thousands of years aromatherapy and massage have been used for medicinal purposes. Natural plant oils have long been recognized for their healing, cleansing, preservative and mood-enhancing properties as well as the sheer pleasure of their fragrances.

This book combines the practice of aromatherapy with the power of touch and massage. With the help of step-by-step pictures and informative text, this volume contains everything you need to know about how to use these soothing arts safely and effectively. You will learn how the oils are produced, which ones you should use and how to benefit from them, by either adding a few drops to your bath or using oil burners to scent the room. You will also discover how to blend oils for massage, the techniques of self-massage, working with a partner, instant massage for stress relief and steps for a healing massage. There are also specific routines that will help you relieve insomnia, alleviate indigestion, soothe headaches and encourage relaxation.

Massage tones the body, stimulates the circulation and releases tension and discomfort. Combined with the powerful, evocative essences of natural plant oils, this restorative therapy has the power to promote physical and emotional balance and well-being.

$\mathscr{A}$ROMATHERAPY

The value of natural plant oils has been recognized for more than 6000 years, because of their healing, cleansing, preservative and mood-enhancing properties, as well as the sheer pleasure of their fragrances. Today, these properties are being rediscovered as we look to the wisdom of past eras and civilizations to restore the balance that has been lost in modern life. Stress, pollution, unhealthy diet, hectic but sedentary lifestyles – all these factors have adverse effects on our bodies and spirits. The art of aromatherapy harnesses the pure essences of aromatic plants, flowers and resins, to work on the most powerful of the senses – smell and touch – to restore the harmony of body and mind. Use the beneficial properties of essential oils to treat common ailments, promote good health and emotional well-being, and to enhance every aspect of your life. These potent, volatile essences are nature's gift to mind and body.

THE HISTORY OF AROMATHERAPY

There is well-documented evidence from the great civilizations of the past to indicate that the use of herbs and aromatics in ancient times was commonplace, and that a large body of knowledge existed concerning the properties of these plants. During the intervening millennia much of this knowledge was lost or ignored, and it is only relatively recently that the wisdom of ancient healers in the application of essential oils has been rediscovered.

DISCOVERING THE SECRETS OF THE OILS

The origins of aromatherapy can be traced through the religious, medical and social practices of all the major civilizations. It is likely that the Chinese were the first to discover the remarkable medicinal powers of plants around 4500 BC. However, it is the Egyptians who must take the credit for recognizing and fully exploiting the physical and spiritual properties of aromatic essences.

From hieroglyphs and tomb paintings we know that aromatic preparations were used as offerings to the gods. Furthermore, the natural antiseptic and bactericidal properties of essential oils and resins, particularly cedarwood and frankincense, made them ideal for the purpose of preserving corpses in preparation for the next world. The discovery of remarkably well-preserved mummies up to 5000 years after their preparation is a tribute to the embalmer's art.

The Egyptians stored their raw materials in large clay or alabaster pots. Water was added and the pots heated so that steam rose and was pushed through a cotton cloth in the neck of the jar. This soaked up the essential oil which was then squeezed and pressed out into a collection vessel. The same principle remains in use in the sophisticated stills employed today.

The back of Tutankhamun's throne shows the King being anointed with perfumed oil by his Queen, Ankhesenamun, 1357–1349 BC.

AROMATICS IN THERAPY

By around 3000 BC Egyptian priests, who had been using the oils in religious ceremonies and embalming rites, became aware of the usefulness of their properties for the living. Closely guarding their secrets, they became the healers of their time, mixing and prescribing "magic" medicinal potions. The use of essential oils gradually permeated all levels of society as cosmetics and perfumes became widespread.

The Chinese, too, used aromatics for religious practices as well as for health, and applied them during massage as an additional means of maintaining a healthy body. The Chinese knowledge of herbs around 2500 BC is documented in *The Yellow Emperor's Classic of Internal Medicine*, traditionally said to have been written by the legendary Emperor Kiwang-Ti. More than 4000 years later in 1579, after 26 years of study, Le Shih-Chên published the Pên T'sao, an enormous and valuable volume in which he recorded the use of 2000 herbs and 20 essential oils. This book documents the greatest range of herbs studied in any tradition.

Many Egyptian paintings show perfume and ointment carriers being used in everyday life.

In ancient Greece the sick were treated with aromatic herbs and spices. Here fragrant herbs are burned in the temple of Asclepius to help a sick child.

In India the traditional Ayervedic medical practice was developed from 2000-year-old texts, which list 700 useful aromatics, all valued for their spiritual and health-giving properties. There, as in China, the principal aspect of this form of medicine was the aromatic massage.

Aromatic substances were among the earliest traded goods, rare and highly prized. Phoenician merchants spread the trade of aromatic material into the Arabian peninsula and across the Mediterranean to Greece and Rome. The Greek physician Marestheus first recorded the stimulating and sedative qualities of different aromatic flowers, and in the first century AD Dioscorides compiled the *Herbarius*, a five-volume study of the sources and uses of plants and aromatics. This became the standard medical treatise for the following thousand years.

The Greeks and Romans used aromatics widely in rituals and ceremonies as well as in medicine, and the oils played an important role in the rise in popularity of baths, massage and body-culture generally throughout the Roman Empire. However, with the fall of the Empire in the fifth century the use of essential oils died out in Europe.

of death among perfumers suggests they were to some degree effective. The fifteenth century saw the rise of the great European perfumers.

Revolutionary developments in science that began during the Renaissance led to the analysis and study of an increasing number of essential oils and other aromatic substances. A famous perfume industry developed in Grasse in the South of France, and by the end of the seventeenth century the distinction between apothecaries, who dealt with herbs for medicinal purposes, and the perfume manufacturers, had become quite pronounced.

A sixteenth-century manuscript showing an alchemist. Much of the European herbalists' lore was adapted from the natural philosophy of the alchemists.

THE DEVELOPMENT OF PERFUMERY

The art flourished elsewhere, though, particularly in Arabia, where Avicenna was the first to distil rose essence around AD 1000. Arabia became the world centre for the production of perfume, importing raw materials from Egypt, India, Tibet and China, and trading its products internationally.

The art of perfumery was reintroduced to Europe at the beginning of the twelfth century with the return of the first Crusaders. Records show that aromatics were used as protection against the plague and the low incidence

Fourteenth-century people had their own herbal lore, and were skilled at gathering and processing certain plants for medical or culinary purposes.

One of the first books on herbalism by John Gerard: these pages show the flower-de-luce.

HERBALISM

The advent of mechanized printing allowed the publication of popular herbals making texts such as Banckes' *Herbal* (1527) available to a wider public. In seventeenth-century England, Nicholas Culpeper, John Parkinson and John Gerard, among others, led the way in the golden age of English herbalism. At the same time, natural philosophy that had been such an important part of the alchemists' work was left behind, to be developed in isolation by artists and thinkers. This development marked the beginning of the separation of body and spirit that is so evident in medical practice today.

During this time, as scientific knowledge about essential oils grew, their use in medicine became less important, and the concept of holism was lost, albeit temporarily. In the mid-seventeenth century the separation between traditional herbalists and physicians who favoured chemical drug therapy began. However, philosophers exploring alchemy further refined the art of distillation, allowing more and more aromatic essences to be created for a wide range of uses.

THE MODERN ART AND PRACTICE OF AROMATHERAPY

The French doctor and scientist René-Maurice Gattefossé is the twentieth-century father of aromatherapy. Gattefossé is credited with coining the name "aromatherapy" to describe treatments with essential oils. His interest was aroused as the result of an accident he sustained while working in the laboratory of a perfumery. He burnt his hand badly and plunged it into the nearest available liquid, which happened to be essential oil of lavender. The burns healed very quickly with minimal scarring, prompting him to research into the healing qualities of this and other essential oils. He also discovered that essential oils are more powerful in their natural state than when their active chemicals are used in isolation. Gattefossé published the results of his findings in his book *Aromathérapie* (1937).

Many of those who came after Gattefossé helped to rediscover the link between the mind and spirit and a healthy body. The Frenchman Jean Valnet, also a doctor and scientist, used essential oils to treat wounds during the Second World War, as well as to treat specific illnesses. Today in France there are many medical doctors prescribing essential oils for internal use to heal ailments.

Valnet's work was taken up and developed by Madame Marguerite Maury, a beauty therapist who was interested in incorporating essential oils into her treatments. Her principle was to revitalize each client by using a personal aromatic blend, which she based on the individual's temperament and specific health disorders.

Madame Maury was dissatisfied with the

Practitioners of the healing arts relied on plants to heal illness for thousands of years. Many of the herbs they commonly used are plants from which essential oils are extracted.

oral administration of essential oils, and rediscovered the method of applying them in diluted form during massage, as had been practised by the ancient healers.

Today, widespread use is made of aromatherapy in many fields of conventional medicine. Aromatherapy has been found to be useful in alleviating the symptoms for patients suffering long-term illnesses such as cancer and AIDS. Most imaginatively, it has recently been used by volunteers working with orphaned children in Romania, and one enterprising South African teacher uses essential oils to create a calm atmosphere of learning and concentration in her township nursery school.

THE ESSENTIAL OILS

An essential oil is the essence or personality of a plant, the plant's life force distilled for use. The fragrance and character of each oil are as individual and unique as a fingerprint, as are its therapeutic properties and the effects they have on the individual. Essential oils are natural, volatile substances that evaporate readily, quickly releasing their aroma into the air, as happens, for example, when someone brushes against an aromatic plant in a garden. The German term for essential oils means "ethereal oils", which is a much more accurate and evocative description. Some 300 essential oils are commercially available, but of these only between 50 and 100 have health-giving properties and are suitable for use in aromatherapy.

SOURCES OF ESSENTIAL OILS

Not all plants contain essential oils. In those that do, the oil, or essence, is contained in highly specialized glands that are present in the foliage, flower or other part of the plant. The purpose of the oil is to help prevent water loss from the plant. As the oils evaporate they create a barrier around the leaf or other part and so reduce evaporation. Essential oils may also provide some defence against infection, and attract insects that are vital to pollination.

The plants that contain essential oils are found mainly in hot, dry habitats. In some plants, such as marjoram, the essential oil glands are present in the minute hairs on the leaves, but in woody plants such as rosewood they are embedded in the fibrous bark or wood. In others the oil glands can be seen clearly as shiny, coloured disks on the surface of the leaf or flower.

At certain times of the day, and particular times of the year, the essential oils are present at optimum levels, and this is the best time for harvest and distillation. The amount of oil produced by a plant is also affected by the growing conditions, including the type of soil, the amount of sunlight it receives, and

French lavender produces a fruitier, sweeter aroma than English lavender, which has a camphorous undertone. It takes 1 tonne/1 ton of plants to yield about 9 kg/20 lb of essential oil.

rainfall. French lavender, for example, is famous for its rich aroma but, like wine, the quality can vary from year to year.

Essential oils have a consistency similar to that of water and most are lighter than water, although some are heavier. All of them differ from vegetable oils in that they are not greasy. Most are colourless; those that are coloured include bergamot, which is green, lemon oil, which is yellow, and chamomile, blue.

Chemical Constituents

A particular oil may contain between 50–500 different chemicals. Rose oil contains the greatest number, some of which are found in such minute quantities that they have not yet been identified. This has made it impossible to reproduce accurately the most exquisite of all essential oils.

Each of the many chemicals present in an essential oil has its own properties, which are in turn imparted to the oil. The chemical complexity of essential oils is responsible for their various characteristics and the actions they produce in the body.

Essential oils evaporate readily: a few drops added to hot water will fragrance a room.

Bottles for essential oils should be of dark glass and have a stopper incorporating a drop dispenser. Keep the bottles tightly closed, and away from direct light and heat.

How Essential Oils Work

Essential oils are composed of tiny molecules which are easily dissolved in alcohol, emulsifiers and, particularly, fats. This allows them to penetrate the skin easily and work into the body by mixing with the fatty tissue.

As these highly volatile essences evaporate they are also inhaled, thus entering the body via the millions of sensitive cells that line the nasal passages. These send messages straight to the brain, and affect the emotions by working on the limbic system, which also controls the major functions of the body.

The chemicals in essential oils unleash the body's ability to heal. They are carried to all parts in the blood, after which they are excreted through the lungs and in the urine. Diluting the oils delays their passage through the body but does not detract from their efficacy. After a treatment, the essential oil remains in the body for 3–4 hours, activating the healing process, which can continue for 2–3 weeks.

Essential oils are able to influence all aspects of the body's functions, from tissues to organs, to body fluids and cells, as well as the emotional state and the spiritual aspects of the person.

Essential oils are used to scent a variety of fragrant objects, such as candles, potpourri and pomanders.

EXTRACTING ESSENTIAL OILS

Most essential oils are produced by distillation or expression. Generally, because of the fragile nature of the raw material, the processing takes place in the country of origin. More robust materials, such as wood, bark, and seeds, are sometimes exported for distillation elsewhere. Herbs and flowers can be distilled fresh or dried, and hardier material such as wood needs to be chipped or even powdered before processing can begin. The citrus oils, contained in the peel of the fruit, are all expressed (squeezed), often by hand. Other essential oils are produced by dry, water or steam distillation.

Distillation

The most common method of production is steam distillation. By this method the volatile and water-soluble parts are separated from the rest of the plant. The resulting mixture may need to be distilled a second time to remove non-volatile matter.

In the distillation process the plant is placed in a sealed container. Water in a second container is heated to produce steam, which is passed under pressure through the plant material. The steam causes the glands containing the essence to burst, allowing the volatile chemicals to dissolve in the steam. This rises and is taken into a condensing chamber, where it is cooled. As it cools and condenses the essential oil is separated from the water. Floral water is a by-product of distilling and, like essential oil, has therapeutic and commercial uses.

Solvent extraction

A lengthier and more expensive process, solvent extraction is favoured for releasing essential oil from more delicate material, such as jasmine flowers. The plant material is washed with a solvent such as alcohol until the essence dissolves. The resulting material is then distilled at a precise, quite low temperature to separate the solvent and the aromatic oil. Oil made by this process is known as an absolute.

The extraction of essential oils from delicate flowers is a time-consuming and costly process.

Store blends of essential and carrier oils in glass bottles, securely stoppered.

BUYING THE FINEST OILS

For the best results use only the finest oils. In general, price is an excellent guide to quality, and it is wise to compare various suppliers' prices so that you can recognize an extremely expensive oil and an unbelievably cheap one. Be aware that essential oils are easily adulterated, and do not be misled by unscrupulous marketing practices. For example, there is no such thing as cheap rose oil; cheap rose oil is probably a similar-smelling product to which geranium or palmarosa oil has been added. Rosemary may also be adulterated, by the addition of camphor or eucalyptus.

If you buy from a reputable source you will also avoid those unscrupulous manufacturers who, although offering a pure essential oil, market oils from a second or third distillation. These will contain only a few active ingredients; the majority will have been removed during the first processing.

Rose is one of the most expensive and complex of all the essential oils.

THE MECHANICS OF SMELLING

When a scent is inhaled, the odour molecules float to the back of the nasal cavity, where they dissolve and unite with receptor, or olfactory, cells. These trigger off electrical signals via the nerve pathways to the olfactory bulb in the brain. Only eight molecules of scent are needed to trigger the smell mechanism. Most of the essential oil molecules that have triggered the system are breathed out, although some will enter the bloodstream via the lungs and will then travel around the body for several hours before they are eliminated.

The areas of the brain to which messages concerning smell are sent are the cerebral cortex and the limbic system. The limbic system controls many vital activities such as sleep, sexual drive, hunger and thirst as well as smell. This is also the area of the brain that

A simple way to enjoy the benefits of an essential oil is to put a drop on a handkerchief.

relates to emotion and memory, which gives the clue to the link between smell, emotion and memory. Odours also connect with the hypothalamus, which controls the endocrine system and nervous system. Through this mechanism the brain comes into contact with the outside world. Specific neuro-chemicals within the nervous system are stimulated by the different scents.

The apparent fading of a scent occurs when all the receptor cells are full, but after ten minutes or so they are vacated and can be reoccupied, causing the scent to "come back". This explains why we fail to notice a scent if we have been exposed to it for a while, while it may smell strong to someone just coming into the room.

A familiar smell has the power to unlock long-lost memories.

Pleasant aromas will have an uplifting effect on your emotional state.

CAUTIONS: Essential oils are highly concentrated substances and must be used with caution. Follow the points listed below and for the treatment of persistent problems, ask the advice of a qualified aromatherapist. If in any doubt, seek a medical opinion before using essential oils.

• Never take essential oils internally, unless professionally prescribed.

• Always use essential oils diluted. Do not exceed the recommended rates: up to 3-6 drops essential oil to 10 ml/2 tsp carrier oil; just 5 drops in a bath or for a steam inhalation.

• Do not use the same oils for more than one or two weeks at any one time.

• When mixing your own blends, do not use more than three oils in any one treatment as the synergistic effects are less predictable.

• Do not use oils in pregnancy without getting professional advice. The following oils are contra-indicated at this time: bay, basil, clary sage, comfrey, fennel, hyssop, juniper, marjoram, melissa, myrrh, rosemary, sage and thyme.

• For anyone with skin problems, dilute the oils even more and, if any skin irritation occurs, stop using them immediately. A few essential oils, such as bergamot, make the skin more sensitive to sunlight, so should be used with caution in hot, sunny weather.

• Be extra careful with anyone who has asthma or epilepsy and if they experience a reaction, stop using the oil.

A fragrance may conjure up a vivid image from the past – perhaps of a secluded garden visited in childhood. Both memory and emotion are linked to our sense of smell; all three are governed by the same area of the brain, the limbic system.

CHOOSING THE RIGHT OILS

The essential oils profiled in the following pages play a major part in the aromatherapist's practice and constitute the principal oils suitable for use in the home. Use the detailed descriptions of their effects to help you choose an oil or put together a blend that will suit your particular needs.

BENZOIN
Styrax benzoin

Benzoin is a warming and comforting oil produced from the sap of a tall tree native to tropical Asia. It is one of the ingredients in Friar's Balsam, a mixture used to treat respiratory complaints. It was also, together with lavender and ethanol, one of the main ingredients in an old-fashioned toilet water called Virgin's Milk, which reputedly left the skin "clear and brilliant". Like sandalwood, it is a traditional ingredient in incense.

APPLICATIONS AND EFFECTS
Calming and soothing. Particularly effective for respiratory conditions and mental and emotional disorders.
Skin: Cracked, dry and chapped skin, also wrinkled skin, chilblains, rashes, wounds, sores, itching; soothing to irritation resulting from sunburn, rashes and hives.
Circulatory and muscular systems: Arthritis, gout, poor circulation, muscular aches and pains, rheumatism.
Respiratory system: Bronchitis (very effective on congested mucous membranes), chills, chesty coughs, sore throats and laryngitis.
Digestive system: Flatulence, colic.
Immune system: 'Flu, cystitis, mouth ulcers.
Nervous system: Insomnia, nervous tension, bed-wetting.
Mental/emotional effects: Calms stress and tension, comforts sad, lonely and depressed individuals. Helps to let go of worries, gives confidence and helps in exhausted emotional and psychic states.

CAUTION: Can cause drowsiness.

BERGAMOT
Citrus bergamia

Bergamot is an ornamental citrus tree native to tropical Asia. The peel of the ripe fruit yields an oil that is mild and gentle, with a sweet, aromatic odour. It is one of the main constituents of eau-de-Cologne and lavender water, and is also found in some sun-tan preparations. The plant is now cultivated in Italy and on the Ivory Coast and its common name may have come from the city of Bergamo in northern Italy. Bergamot leaves are used to flavour Earl Grey tea. Not to be confused with the herb bergamot (*Monarda didyma*).

APPLICATIONS AND EFFECTS
Particularly effective for boils, eczema, psoriasis, anxiety and depression.
Skin: Acne, cold sores, insect bites, insect repellent, oily complexions (especially stress-related), spots, wounds.
Respiratory system: Bad breath, sore throat, tonsillitis, bronchitis.
Digestive system: Flatulence, poor appetite (has a regulating action, which may be useful for anorexia), colic, indigestion.
Reproductive and excretory systems: Cystitis, thrush.
Nervous system: PMS (mood swings), insomnia, nightmares.
Immune system: Colds, 'flu, fever, cold sores, chicken pox, immune deficiency, herpes.
Mental/emotional effects: Its cooling and refreshing action helps soothe anger and frustration. Bergamot is useful for grief; the uplifting nature of this oil makes the bereaved receptive to joy and love again.

CAUTION: Not to be used before going out into the sun, even when diluted, as it can cause discoloration of the skin that results in a rash.

BLACK PEPPER
Piper nigrum

The essential oil of black pepper comes from the fruit of a tropical vine. These fruits are the same peppercorns used for culinary purposes, the familiar spice commonly added to food. The vine, which has heart-shaped leaves and white blooms, is extensively cultivated in South-east Asia. Black pepper is one of the three oldest-known spices, the other two being cloves and cinnamon. The oil is warming and comforting and surprisingly sweet; it can often add a mysterious depth to a blend. In ancient times it was very highly valued: it is said of Attila the Hun that he demanded black pepper as part of the ransom for Rome.

APPLICATIONS AND EFFECTS

Particularly effective for muscular aches and pains, fevers, colds, 'flu.
Skin: Chilblains.
Circulatory and muscular systems: Arthritis, neuralgia, poor circulation, rheumatic pain, sprains, stiffness, poor muscle tone.
Respiratory system: Catarrh, chills. Used as a homeopathic remedy, it can relieve fevers.
Digestive system: Colic, constipation, sluggish digestion, diarrhoea, flatulence, heartburn, loss of appetite, nausea.
Immune system: Colds, 'flu, infections caused by bacteria (urinary, respiratory or digestive), viral infections.
Mental/emotional effects: Gives stamina where there is frustration, and enthusiasm where there is indifference. Can help where there is lack of interest and vitality, such as when recovering from an infection.

CAUTION: Care should be taken by those with sensitive skins, as in high concentrations it can occasionally cause irritation. Too frequent use may over-stimulate the kidneys.

CEDARWOOD
Cedrus atlantica

Cedar is a Semitic word meaning "the power of spiritual strength". The tree from which the essential oil is extracted is native to the Atlas mountains of Morocco, but it is now grown more widely, particularly in Lebanon and some parts of the Far East. The majestically tall, pyramid-shaped evergreen gives an oil that embodies the ancient qualities of its name – confidence and firmly rooted spiritual strength. The oil is extracted by steam distillation from the wood of the tree. It was used in ancient times by the Egyptians in the form of a gum, as a main ingredient for the preservation of mummies, and it is thought to be one of the earliest-known oils. The oil is still used by Tibetans as a temple incense and by natives of North Africa for medicinal purposes.

APPLICATIONS AND EFFECTS

Particularly effective for long-standing complaints rather than acute ones; has aphrodisiac properties.
Skin: Acne, dandruff.
Circulatory and muscular systems: Arthritis, rheumatism, poor circulation.
Respiratory system: Bronchitis, catarrh, coughs, chest infections.
Reproductive and excretory systems: Cystitis.
Mental/emotional effects: This uplifting oil is useful for lack of confidence or fearfulness. It has euphoric properties that help to eliminate mental stagnation in depressed states. It is relaxing and soothing and can be a good aid to meditation.

CAUTION: Best avoided during pregnancy.

CHAMOMILE
Anthemis nobilis

There is a long tradition of use for this gentle yet strengthening herb. The Moors and Egyptians recognized its calming qualities and the Saxons used it as part of their mixture of nine sacred herbs in an incense known as "maythen". There are several varieties of chamomile from which essential oils are obtained, but the most commonly used are Roman chamomile (*Anthemis nobilis*) and German chamomile (*Matricaria chamomilla*). They have similar properties, although they differ in appearance. Roman chamomile is a creeping perennial with tiny, needle-like leaves; German chamomile is a taller, upright annual with fragile, feathery leaves. Both have small, white, daisy-like flowers. The essential oil of German chamomile has a larger proportion of the anti-inflammatory chemical azulene, which is useful for treating skin conditions.

APPLICATIONS AND EFFECTS

Calming. Particularly effective for teething pain, headaches.

Skin: Acne, allergies, boils, burns, chilblains, earache, inflammations, insect bites, toothache.

Circulatory and muscular systems: Arthritis, muscular pain, rheumatism, sprains.

Digestive system: Colic, indigestion, nausea.

Reproductive and excretory systems: Painful periods, menopause, PMS, cystitis.

Immune system: Thrush, fever.

Nervous system: Insomnia, nervous tension, bed-wetting.

Mental/emotional effects: A gently sedative oil for the highly strung and over-enthusiastic. Useful where symptoms are related to anger, irritability or unexpressed emotions.

CAUTION: Some people may find it causes dermatitis.

CLARY SAGE
Salvia sclarea

This tall, biennial herb grows in most parts of the world and provides a powerful aromatic, yet benevolent, euphoric oil. Its leaves are rather similar to those of common sage, although they are broader, wrinkled and hairy. The blue-white flowers are smaller than those of the more familiar herb and are enclosed in greeny-yellow, sometimes purplish, bracts. The Latin name *salvia* means "good health" and *sclarea* means "clear". Because of its euphoric properties it was sometimes substituted for hops in the brewing of beer. Today it is more widely used as a culinary herb in soups and stews as well as in the perfume industry.

APPLICATIONS AND EFFECTS

Particularly effective for reproductive and excretory disorders.

Skin: Acne, boils, dandruff.

Circulatory and muscular systems: High blood pressure, muscular aches and pains.

Respiratory system: Throat infections.

Digestive system: Colic, cramp, flatulence.

Reproductive and excretory systems: Irregular or painful periods, PMS, menopausal problems.

Immune system: Myalgic encephalomyelitis (ME), convalescence.

Nervous system: Depression, migraine, nervous tension, insomnia, panic.

Mental/emotional effects: Useful for difficulty in adjusting to change. Helps put things into perspective. Encourages dream recall; may help the individual to see more clearly.

CAUTION: Should be avoided by pre-menopausal women with a history of breast, cervical, ovarian or uterine cancer. May cause problems in some women taking the contraceptive pill or hormone replacement therapy (HRT). Avoid using with alcohol as it may exaggerate the effects or cause nausea. Not to be used before driving.

CYPRESS
Cupressus sempervirens

The cypress tree is a statuesque evergreen that grows wild in southern France, Italy, Spain, Portugal, Corsica and North Africa. The specific Latin name *sempervirens* means "everlasting", and both the Egyptians and Romans dedicated it to their deities of the underworld. The essential oil is yellow and has a rich scent similar to the scent of pine needles. It is extracted from the cones of the plant by steam distillation; the main centres of production are in Europe, in Germany and France.

APPLICATIONS AND EFFECTS

Useful when there is an excess of fluids in some way. Particularly effective for diarrhoea, water retention and runny colds.

Skin: Oily and puffy skin, sweaty feet (when blended with peppermint), wounds.

Circulatory and muscular systems: Cellulite, muscular cramps, poor circulation, rheumatism.

Respiratory system: Bronchitis, spasmodic coughing, 'flu.

Digestive system: Haemorrhoids.

Reproductive and excretory systems: Heavy and painful periods, menopausal problems, cystitis.

Nervous system: Nervous tension.

Mental/emotional effects: The solemn nature of cypress makes it useful during periods of transition such as bereavement. It is also helpful at times for feelings of sadness and self-pity. It can be useful for soothing anger and quietening over-talkative people. It is spiritually cleansing and aids the removal of psychic blocks.

CAUTION: Should be used with caution during pregnancy.

EUCALYPTUS
Eucalyptus globulus

Some 15 species of this tall evergreen tree yield a useful essential oil. They include *Eucalyptus citriadoria* and *E. radiata*, as well as *E. globulus*. The leaves and oil of the plant have long been a household remedy in Australia, where the aborigines, who know it as "kino", use it to dress wounds. The young trees, which have round, bluish leaves, are valued by florists and gardeners. As the plants mature the foliage becomes long, narrow and yellowish in colour. The flowers are white and the smooth bark is often covered with a white bloom.

APPLICATIONS AND EFFECTS

Useful in congested and toxic states. Particularly effective for muscular aches, bronchitis, colds, coughs, sinusitis and throat infections.

Skin: Insect bites, insect repellent.

Circulatory and muscular systems: Poor circulation, arthritis.

Reproductive and excretory systems: Cystitis, diarrhoea.

Nervous system: Headaches.

Immune system: 'Flu, fevers.

Mental/emotional effects: This oil has a deeply grounding quality, which can help cool overheated emotions. Its cleansing and harmonizing nature makes it useful where there has been emotional or physical conflict, and for places that just feel uncomfortable. It may also aid concentration.

CAUTION: Some people may find it irritates the skin.

FRANKINCENSE
Boswellia thurifera

Frankincense (also known as olibanum) is an inspiring and contemplative oil that comes from the gum of a small tree or shrub grown mainly in the Middle East, with most of the oil produced in Iran and Lebanon. The gum is extracted by incising the trunk and peeling away the bark. The oozing juice slowly hardens on contact with the air and is then collected for distillation. The gum was highly prized in ancient times and was known simply by the old French name *franc encens*, "frank" meaning high quality. Frankincense is familiar primarily from its biblical connection as one of the three gifts to the infant Jesus: at that time its value was almost as great as that of gold. In ancient Egypt it was used as an incense in religious ceremonies and in cosmetics, where it was valued for its rejuvenating properties.

APPLICATIONS AND EFFECTS

Particularly effective for mature skin, bronchitis and anxiety.
Skin: Dry skin, scars, wounds, sores, ulcers.
Respiratory system: Catarrh, coughs, laryngitis, rheumatic conditions.
Reproductive and excretory systems: Cystitis, painful periods, heavy periods.
Immune system: Colds, 'flu.
Nervous system: Nervous tension, fear, nightmares.
Mental/emotional effects: Regulating oil, yet stimulating. This makes it useful in cases of exhaustion and mental fatigue. Useful for those who lack confidence and are weary of spirit. An excellent aid to meditation, as it deepens and slows the breath.

GERANIUM
Pelargonium graveolens

This adaptable oil has been widely used since antiquity, when it was thought to keep evil spirits at bay. The essential oil is strong when pure but sweetens when diluted. It comes from a perennial shrub covered in tiny hairs, which bears small pink flowers and has pointed, serrated leaves from which the essential oil is obtained, though all parts of the plant are scented. The plant is native to Africa, but is now cultivated in many parts of the world, as a house plant as well as commercially for its oil. Production of the oil is centred mainly in Réunion; other producers include France, Italy, China and Egypt.

APPLICATIONS AND EFFECTS

Particularly effective for sluggish, oily complexions and combination skin, irregular menstrual periods, mood swings and post-natal depression.
Skin: Acne, bruises, burns, chilblains, dermatitis, eczema, herpes, wounds.
Circulatory and muscular systems: Cellulite, poor circulation, fluid retention, detoxifying the body.
Respiratory system: Sore throats, tonsillitis.
Reproductive and excretory systems: PMS, menopause, urinary infections.
Nervous system: Nervous tension, diarrhoea resulting from a nervous condition, anxiety, depression.
Mental/emotional effects: Balancing, harmonizing and cleansing. Can be stimulating and uplifting. A useful alternative to bergamot as an anti-depressant oil.

GINGER
Zingiber officinale

Like benzoin, the essential oil of ginger is known for its warm, comforting nature. The oil is extracted from the dried tuberous root of a plant that is native to south Asia. The plant itself has a reed-like stalk with narrow, spear-shaped leaves and yellow or white flowers that are carried on a spike rising straight from the tuber. There is some debate as to the derivation of its name. The Greeks called it *ziggiber*, and in Sanskrit writings it is listed as *srngavera*. However, its name may come from the area called Gingi, where it was drunk as a tea to cure stomachache.

APPLICATIONS AND EFFECTS

Quintessentially balancing; counteracts ailments caused by dampness. Particularly effective for muscular aches and pains, catarrh, coughs and colds (especially runny colds).
Skin: Clears bruises.
Circulatory and muscular systems: Poor circulation, rheumatism, sprains, strains.
Respiratory system: Congestion, sinusitis, chills.
Digestive system: Diarrhoea, colic, cramp, flatulence, indigestion, hangovers, loss of appetite, nausea, travel sickness.
Reproductive and excretory systems: Regulates menstruation after colds.
Immune system: Fever, 'flu, infectious disease, sore throat.
Nervous system: Debility, nervous exhaustion or fatigue.
Mental/emotional effects: This oil is comforting and grounding at the same time. When emotions are flat and cold it can be used to warm them. Ginger sharpens the senses and memory.

CAUTION: May be slightly phototoxic. In high concentrations it may cause skin irritation.

GRAPEFRUIT
Citrus paradisi

The grapefruit tree is cultivated for its delicious, large, yellow fruits. The tree reaches about 10 m/33 ft in height, and bears dark, glossy leaves and white flowers. It is native to tropical Asia and the West Indies, although it probably originated in Asia as a hybrid of the orange tree. Grapefruit trees are grown as ornamental trees all over the Mediterranean and are also cultivated in Florida, Brazil and Israel. California is the main producer of the oil. The yield of oil from the fresh peel is small when compared to the yields from the orange and lemon. Like other citrus oils it has a relatively short shelf life.

APPLICATIONS AND EFFECTS

Cleansing, balancing, brightening and refreshing. Particularly effective for congested pores and oily skin, cellulite, and the digestion of fatty foods.
Skin: Acne.
Circulatory and muscular systems: Muscle fatigue, exercise preparation, stiffness, water retention, migraine.
Digestive system: Loss of appetite, cleansing the kidneys, liver tonic.
Reproductive and excretory systems: PMS.
Immune system: Chills, colds, flu.
Nervous system: Depression, headaches, migraine, performance stress, nervous exhaustion, jet lag, restoration of balance after ear infections.
Mental/emotional effects: Use this uplifting oil when feeling apathetic or indecisive. Its euphoric nature may help with feelings of resentfulness, jealousy and envy.

CAUTION: Presents a very slight risk of producing photosensitivity in the skin.

JASMINE
Jasminum officinale

Described as "the king of flower oils" and "the scent of angels", jasmine is renowned as an aphrodisiac and is often used in love potions. It is a tall evergreen vine with bright green leaves and highly fragrant, white, star-shaped flowers. The flowers are harvested at night in order to obtain the most intense aroma. In India guests are often welcomed with garlands of the flowers. Jasmine is popular as a flavouring for tea in China; and in Europe it is used medicinally. The plant is grown in many parts of the world, including the Middle East, China, North Africa, France and Italy.

APPLICATIONS AND EFFECTS

It has a strong, masculine scent and produces feelings of optimism, euphoria and confidence.

Skin: Dry, greasy, irritated or sensitive skin (but see caution, below).

Circulatory and muscular systems: Muscular spasm, sprains.

Respiratory system: Catarrh, coughs, laryngitis, hoarseness.

Reproductive and excretory systems: PMS, painful periods; promotes labour and lactation.

Nervous system: Depression, nervous exhaustion.

Mental/emotional effects: This emotionally warming oil has the ability to unite the opposing factors within us. It is most useful at times when there is apathy, indifference, and coldness.

CAUTION: Generally safe to use, although some individuals may have an allergic reaction to it. It can give some people a headache and its narcotic quality may impede concentration.

JUNIPER
Juniperus communis

This evergreen tree or shrub has fine, stiff, needle-like leaves of bluish-green and small flowers that are followed by tiny berries. The tree is native to Scandinavia, Siberia, Canada, northern Europe, and Asia. Its medicinal properties are known throughout the world. The Greeks, Romans, and Arabs valued its antiseptic properties, while the Mongolians used it to assist women in labour. More recently, juniper and rosemary have been burned to clear the air in French hospitals. In the Bible, Elijah sleeps under a juniper tree (Kings 1:19:4–5), connecting it with the ability to revive the spirits.

APPLICATIONS AND EFFECTS

Its most important use is as a detoxifier. Also particularly effective for cellulite, absence of menstrual periods, cystitis, water retention and painful periods.

Skin: Acne, dermatitis, eczema, haemorrhoids, toner for oily skin, wounds.

Circulatory and muscular systems: Toxic states generally, gout, arthritis, cramps, rheumatism.

Digestive system: Detoxifying.

Immune system: Colds, 'flu, coughs, purification of the blood, useful following infection.

Nervous system: Anxiety, nervous tension.

Mental/emotional effects: Strengthens the spirit and purifies the atmosphere. Can help in challenging situations and when overcome with feelings of regret for past actions.

CAUTION: Some people may find it irritating, and it is best avoided during pregnancy. Not to be used by people with kidney disease.

LAVENDER
Lavandula angustifolia/officinalis

Lavender has been the most popular essential oil for centuries. The plant is an easily recognized evergreen shrub with narrow, pale silver-green leaves and spikes of flowers ranging in colour from pink and white to pale or deep blue. It is widely cultivated in France, Bulgaria and England. Lavender was used by the Romans to bathe in and to cleanse wounds. In England it was commonly used to scent linen boxes, as an aid to controlling insects. Lavender water was the favourite perfume of Queen Henrietta Maria, wife of Charles I of England, and her partiality was responsible for it becoming popular and fashionable.

APPLICATIONS AND EFFECTS
Mellow, peaceful and the most versatile of all the essential oils. Particularly useful for burns, stress headaches and insomnia.
Skin: Sunburn, bruises, earache, insect bites, cuts.
Circulatory and muscular systems: Muscular aches and painful rheumatism.
Digestive system: Nausea, vomiting, flatulence, indigestion.
Reproductive and excretory systems: Painful and scanty periods.
Immune system: 'Flu, colds, myalgic encephalomyelitis (ME).
Nervous system: Stress headaches, insomnia, shock, vertigo.
Mental/emotional effects: Gently sedative, its balancing action makes it useful for panic states, or impatience and anger. Lavender cleanses both physically and spiritually. It aids in breaking bad habits and is soothing during a crisis.

LEMON
Citrus limonum

The lemon tree is native to Asia, although it now grows wild in the Mediterranean, particularly in Spain and Portugal. It is cultivated extensively in many parts of the world, including North and South America, Israel, Guinea, Cyprus, Sicily and Italy. The tree grows to only 2 m/6 ft in height; it is evergreen with small serrated oval leaves and highly fragrant pink or white flowers. The fruits ripen from green to yellow. The oil was used by the ancient Egyptians as an antidote to food poisoning, and to cure epidemics of fever. In most European countries it was regarded as a cure, but its main use was as a treatment for infectious disease.

APPLICATIONS AND EFFECTS
Fresh, strong and versatile, it harmonizes well and adds character. Particularly effective for arthritis, rheumatism, cellulite, nausea, diarrhoea and haemorrhoids.
Skin: Acne, brittle nails, boils, chilblains, greasy skin, cold sores, insect bites, mouth ulcers, spots, warts, verrucas, bruises.
Circulatory and muscular systems: Nosebleeds, congestion, poor circulation, muscular aches and pains.
Respiratory system: Throat infections, bronchitis, catarrh, sinusitis.
Digestive system: Indigestion, flatulence, heartburn, constipation.
Nervous system: Headaches, migraine.
Immune system: Colds, 'flu, fever, coughs, infections (chronic and recurrent), candida, allergies.
Mental/emotional effects: Can help refresh and clarify thought. Good for feelings of bitterness or resentment about life's injustices, and useful when someone is feeling touchy or when begrudging others' good fortune and success.

CAUTION: May sensitize the skin in some people. Use with caution when sunbathing as it may cause skin discoloration and rash.

MANDARIN
Citrus reticulata

The fruit of the mandarin tree was the ancient and traditional gift to the mandarins of China, where the plant is a native species. It is an evergreen tree with shiny leaves, fragrant white flowers and juicy, edible fruit. The tree was introduced to Europe at the beginning of the nineteenth century, and some 40 years later into the United States. The Americans renamed the tree and fruit the tangerine, but the latter is in fact a larger and rounder fruit with a more yellow skin than the mandarin. The mandarin is grown in Italy, Spain, Algeria, Cyprus, Greece, the Middle East and Brazil.

APPLICATIONS AND EFFECTS

Refined, soft, cheerful, uplifting, sweet. Particularly effective for congested pores and oily skin, and fluid retention.

Skin: Acne, spots, stretch marks.

Circulatory and muscular systems: Helps to tone and improve the circulation.

Digestive system: Digestive problems, pain, flatulence, heartburn, nausea, hiccups.

Nervous system: Insomnia, restlessness, nervous tension.

Mental/emotional effects: This is a balancing oil that can be relaxing or a tonic, according to the individual's needs. It is good for dejected spirits and feelings of emotional emptiness, or the regretting of the passage of time and past losses. It is uplifting, and brings the message of happiness to children. It also helps adults make contact with their own inner child.

CAUTION: Generally safe to use but, like other citrus oils, it should be used with caution in the sun and under other sources of ultraviolet light.

MARJORAM
Origanum majorana

Marjoram is a small perennial plant with hairy stems and dark green, oval leaves. It is native to the Mediterranean region and North Africa, and was often planted in graveyards to bring peace to the departed spirits. The Latin name may be derived from *maior*, meaning "greater", not because there is a lesser variety, but in the sense of conferring longevity. The species name is derived from two Greek words, *oros* and *ganos*, which together mean "joy of the mountains". The herb is used extensively in cooking. The essential oil is extracted from the leaves; it has a very bitter taste and a refined fragrance.

APPLICATIONS AND EFFECTS

Gentle, warming and comforting. Particularly effective for constipation, flatulence, menstrual disorders, anxiety, tension, panic and insomnia.

Skin: Chilblains, bruises.

Circulatory and muscular systems: Arthritis, muscular aches and stiffness, rheumatism, sprains, strains.

Respiratory system: Bronchitis, coughs.

Digestive system: Colic.

Reproductive and excretory systems: PMS.

Immune system: Colds.

Nervous system: Headaches.

Mental/emotional effects: A sedative oil and aphrodisiac. Helpful in highly excitable states and may be useful for hyperactive children. Strengthens the mind and aids in confronting difficult issues such as recent grief.

CAUTION: Best avoided during pregnancy.

NEROLI
Citrus aurantium

The evergreen tree from which the essential oil is produced is native to China, where it was used by traditional Chinese herbalists. The expressed oil is produced in Israel, Cyprus, Brazil and North America. It is a less robust and smaller plant than the bitter orange variety and without the spiny branches or the heart-shaped leaves. The flowers were traditionally used in wedding bouquets to symbolize innocence and to secure love. Orange flower water features in Eastern European cookery and is an ingredient in eau-de-Cologne, which was very popular with those Victorian ladies frequently overcome with the "vapours". Neroli is one of the finest of the floral essences.

APPLICATIONS AND EFFECTS
Simple happiness; nourishing to the soul. Particularly effective for nervous diarrhoea and stress-related conditions.
Skin: Dull, oily, dry and sensitive skin, mouth ulcers, broken veins.
Circulatory and muscular systems: Palpitations, poor circulation.
Respiratory system: Bronchitis, chills.
Digestive system: Constipation, indigestion, flatulence, nausea.
Nervous system: Nervous tension, headaches and insomnia.
Immune system: Colds, 'flu.
Mental/emotional effects: Hypnotic and euphoric. Gives a feeling of peace; useful during times of anxiety, panic, hysteria or shock and fear. Invaluable for soothing when difficulties stem from a relationship. It can help in the development of self-esteem and self-love, comfort the sad, and bring people into contact with their feminine aspect.

CAUTION: The distilled oil is phototoxic, but the expressed oil is not. Generally safe to use although some individuals may get dermatitis.

NUTMEG
Myristica fragrans

Nutmeg and mace are most widely used as culinary spices both in the East and West. The fruit is like a small peach of which the nutmeg is the seed, contained in a bright red husk. Mace, the husk, is used independently as a milder spice than nutmeg. The tree is cultivated in Indonesia, Sri Lanka and the West Indies – particularly Grenada – and the oil is distilled in Europe and the United States. Nutmeg oil has been used in diverse ways, for example in Malaysia as a tonic for pregnant women, and in the manufacture of candles and soap. The Egyptians used it in embalming and in Italy it was an ingredient in incense, used to give protection against the plague.

APPLICATIONS AND EFFECTS
Particularly effective for muscular aches and pains, poor circulation, sluggish digestion, loss of appetite and the early stages of a cold.
Circulatory and muscular systems: Arthritis, gout, rheumatism.
Digestive system: Flatulence, indigestion, nausea, constipation.
Immune system: Bacterial infection, convalescence.
Nervous system: Nervous fatigue.
Mental/emotional effects: This oil is warming, stimulating and a euphoric. It can be comforting to those who find themselves physically and emotionally isolated, such as the elderly.

CAUTION: Use in moderation and with care during pregnancy.

ORANGE
Citrus aurantium

The essential oil called orange and the preserve, marmalade, come from the small, bitter fruit known as the Seville orange, which differs from the familiar, edible, sweet orange, *Citrus sinensis*. *C. aurantium* has shiny, dark green, oval leaves that are pale beneath; the smooth, grey-green branches have long, blunt spines and the small, white flowers are highly fragrant. The plant has become a symbol of both innocence and fertility. The Crusaders brought it back to Europe with them from North Africa and early missionaries introduced it into California. The United States is now one of the main producers of the oil. Because the oil oxidizes very quickly it cannot be kept for very long.

APPLICATIONS AND EFFECTS

Mellow, warming and soothing. Has similar properties to neroli and can be used in similar conditions.

Skin: Dull and oily complexions, mouth ulcers.
Circulatory and muscular systems: Muscular aches and pains, water retention, detoxifying.
Respiratory system: Bronchitis, chills.
Digestive system: Constipation, colic, indigestion (aids digestion of fats), diarrhoea, stimulates appetite.
Immune system: Colds, 'flu, fevers.
Nervous system: Nervous tension, insomnia due to anxiety.
Mental/emotional effects: Lifts gloomy thoughts and depression and encourages a positive outlook. Useful for replenishing cheerfulness. Revives the spirit when it is lacking in energy and relieves boredom. Quells "butterflies" in the stomach.

CAUTION: Generally safe to use, although, like other citrus oils, it increases the photosensitivity of the skin and can cause irritation under ultraviolet light, particularly from the sun. Occasionally causes dermatitis.

PALMAROSA
Cymbopogon martini

This herbaceous plant is native to India and Pakistan, but is cultivated in parts of Africa, in Indonesia, the Comoro Islands and Brazil. Palmarosa has fine, elegant stems and bears flowers on the tip of each stem. The oil is extracted from the leaves. At one time it was exported from the sub-continent and shipped from Bombay to the Red Sea ports. From there it was taken overland to Istanbul (then Constantinople) and to Bulgaria, where it was used to adulterate the highly prized rose oil known as attar of roses, gaining the name "Indian" or "Turkish" oil.

APPLICATIONS AND EFFECTS

Gentle and comforting. Particularly effective for skin inflammations, scars, weak digestion and headaches.

Skin: Acne, dermatitis, minor skin infections, scars, sores; all skin types.
Circulatory and muscular systems: Rheumatic conditions.
Respiratory system: Palpitations.
Digestive system: Intestinal infections.
Reproductive and excretory systems: Candida, cystitis.
Immune system: Myalgic encephalomyelitis (ME).
Nervous system: Nervous exhaustion.
Mental/emotional effects: This is a refreshing oil that can be an aid to spiritual healing. Its cooling quality is useful for anger, jealousy, irritability, hot-headedness and burning, passionate feelings.

PEPPERMINT
Mentha piperita

Peppermint is a perennial herb that is cultivated throughout the world. White peppermint has green stems and leaves, the black variety has dark green, serrated leaves, purplish stems and reddish-violet flowers. Legend relates how Mentha, a nymph pursued by Hades, was trampled into the ground by Hades' jealous wife, Persephone. Out of compassion for her treatment, Hades transformed Mentha into the herb. Peppermint's medicinal qualities were widely appreciated by the ancient Egyptians, Chinese and Indians. The Romans used to crown themselves with peppermint wreaths during feasts, in order to take advantage of its detoxifying effects.

APPLICATIONS AND EFFECTS
Particularly useful for muscular aches and pains, sore feet, headache, indigestion and flatulence, stomach cramps, nausea, colds, fevers.
Skin: Acne, dermatitis, toothache.
Circulatory and muscular systems: Palpitations.
Respiratory system: Bronchitis.
Digestive system: Morning and travel sickness, bad breath.
Immune system: 'Flu, sinusitis.
Mental/emotional effects: Useful for mental fatigue and as an aid to clear thinking. Helpful for anger or hysteria, nervous trembling, shyness and hyper-sensitivity. Overcomes feelings of inferiority by dispelling pride. Associated with cleanliness and the wish to live ethically.

CAUTION: Can be a slight irritant for sensitive skins. May counteract the effects of homeopathic remedies, and suppress milk flow in breast-feeding mothers. Too much in the evenings may cause disturbed sleep patterns.

ROSE
Rosa × damascena trigintipetala

The fresh rose petals used to produce the essential oil are harvested early in the morning just after the dew has settled, and distilled immediately to maximize the yield. The finest oil – the famous and extremely expensive attar of roses – comes from an area in Bulgaria, lying halfway between Sofia and the Black Sea, known as the Valley of Roses. Other roses used in the production of rose oil include *Rosa centifolia*, or the Provence rose. These are also cultivated in Grasse, the centre of the perfume industry in the South of France.

APPLICATIONS AND EFFECTS
Promotes a feeling of well-being and the development of tolerance. Particularly effective for mature skin and stomach upsets with an emotional origin.
Skin: Broken veins, conjunctivitis, dry skin, eczema, sensitive skin.
Circulatory and muscular systems: Palpitations, poor circulation.
Respiratory system: Coughs, allergies affecting the lungs.
Digestive system: Liver congestion (caused by a surplus of blood), nausea, constipation.
Reproductive and excretory systems: Irregular and painful periods.
Nervous system: Depression, insomnia, headache, nervous tension.
Mental/emotional effects: Loneliness, grief and past emotional trauma, such as repressed anger or problems in relationships, can all be helped by this euphoric oil. Useful when dealing with bitter feelings such as jealousy or smouldering anger. Helps people make a fresh start, as it is emotionally healing and cleansing.

ROSEMARY
Rosmarinus officinalis

Rosemary is a shrubby evergreen bush cultivated in most parts of the world, but native to the Mediterranean region. It has scented, silver-grey, needle-like leaves and pale lilac or blue flowers, from which the oil is distilled. In ancient Greece it was burned in shrines, and in ancient Rome it was regarded as a symbol of regeneration. The Moors planted it around their orchards as an insect repellent and it was used in the Middle Ages as a fumigant to drive away evil spirits. More recently, the French used it as a disinfectant in hospital wards during epidemics.

APPLICATIONS AND EFFECTS

Vigorous, penetrating and stimulating. Particularly effective as a remedy for fluid retention and muscular pain.

Skin: Acne, dandruff, dermatitis, eczema, greasy hair, insect repellent.

Circulatory and muscular systems: Gout, palpitations, poor circulation, rheumatism.

Respiratory system: Bronchitis.

Digestive system: Flatulence, indigestion.

Reproductive and excretory systems: Painful menstrual periods.

Nervous system: Debility, headaches, high blood pressure, mental fatigue, nervous exhaustion.

Mental/emotional effects: It can be useful for mental fatigue or lethargy, poor memory or confusion. Rosemary strengthens the mind where there is weakness and exhaustion, and can be used when feeling apathetic or desiring to escape. It is a psychic protector for both individuals and places.

CAUTION: Should be avoided in pregnancy and by epileptics, and used with caution by those with sensitive skins.

SANDALWOOD
Santalum album

Sandalwood has a persistent, sensuous perfume and is one of the oldest-known scented materials, with perhaps as many as 4000 years of uninterrupted use. The essential oil of *Santalum album* is distilled from the heartwood of 30- to 60-year-old evergreen trees growing in Mysore, India. Because the wood is resistant to ant infestation, it was used in the construction of both furniture and buildings, a use that eventually resulted in near extinction of the species. Export of the wood is now illegal and all trees are owned by the Indian government. Oils originating from countries other than India are far inferior in quality.

APPLICATIONS AND EFFECTS

Gentle and sedative. Particularly effective for acne, dry and oily skins, persistent coughs, cystitis, stress and fear.

Skin: Dehydrated, cracked or chapped skin, barber's rash, itching, inflammation, dry eczema, boils, cuts and wounds.

Respiratory system: Bronchitis, catarrh, dry coughs, laryngitis, sore throat.

Immune system: Immune system booster for persistent conditions.

Nervous system: Depression, insomnia, diarrhoea caused by nervous conditions, paranoia; a sensual stimulant.

Mental/emotional effects: Can help encourage self-expression and boost lack of confidence. Brings peace and acceptance, and is therefore useful for grieving, helping the individual cut their ties with the past. Creates a balance for possessive and manipulative people who have difficulty in forgiving. Quietens mental chatter while meditating, allowing deeper meditative states to be reached; useful for healing and self-healing.

CAUTION: May sometimes cause contact dermatitis.

TEA TREE
Melaleuca alternifolia

The tea tree is native to Australia, and is cultivated for its oil along the coast of New South Wales. It has narrow leaves and bears yellow or purple flowers. The essential oil is one of only a few that have been extensively studied. The results revealed that tea tree oil is active against all types of infectious organisms: bacteria, fungi and viruses. It is also a very powerful immune stimulant, increasing the body's ability to respond to these organisms. The oil was a component of tropical first-aid kits during the Second World War, but as antibiotics were developed it was dropped from use, only to be rediscovered as aromatherapy has gained in popularity.

APPLICATIONS AND EFFECTS

Particularly effective in fighting infectious organisms.
Skin: Abscess, acne, athlete's foot, blisters, cold sores, dandruff, dry scalp, insect bites, rashes (nappy rash), spots, verrucas, warts, infected wounds.
Respiratory system: Bronchitis, catarrh, coughs, sinusitis, throat infections, ear infections.
Reproductive and excretory systems: Thrush, cystitis.
Immune system: Colds, fevers, 'flu, infectious diseases including chicken-pox, systemic candida, mouth ulcers, myalgic encephalomyelitis (ME), post-operative shock, reducing the risk of infection, boosting the immune system in convalescence.
Nervous system: The oil is vigorous and revitalizing, and is particularly useful after shock. It is also very refreshing.

CAUTION: Some individuals may develop a sensitivity to it.

YLANG YLANG
Cananga odorata

The name ylang ylang means "flower of flowers", and the very fragrant plant is sometimes called "poor man's jasmine". The source of this essential oil is a beautiful evergreen tree native to Madagascar and the Philippines. It is now cultivated in several parts of the world, including Sumatra, Java and the Comoros. The oil comes from the tree's delicate yellow flowers, which have a very sweet scent reminiscent of almonds and jasmine. Many different qualities of oil are available; the finest is said to come from the flowers of trees grown in Réunion and picked in early morning at the beginning of summer. In Indonesia the voluptuously fragrant flowers are ceremonially scattered on the beds of newly married couples. The essential oil is widely used in perfumes and other aromatic products.

APPLICATIONS AND EFFECTS

Particularly effective for accelerated breathing and palpitations, insomnia and bowel infections.
Skin: Combination skin.
Circulatory and muscular systems: High blood pressure.
Digestive system: Gastro-enteritis.
Nervous system: Depression, anxiety.
Mental/emotional effects: This exotic, luxurious oil creates a feeling of peace and dispels anger, especially anger born of frustration. Its voluptuous nature is reassuring and builds confidence.

CAUTION: Some people may feel headachy or nauseous after using the oil, especially if it is used in concentrated form.

OILS FOR COMMON PROBLEMS

KEY
R Relaxing oil
S Stimulating oil
U Uplifting oil

Some oils have more than one of these properties, tending to balance or normalize the emotions and bodily systems.

CAUTION: This chart is a general guide only. For the treatment of persistent problems, seek the advice of a qualified aromatherapist. Chronic conditions should be referred to a medical practitioner.

Never mix more than three oils in any one treatment as the synergistic effects are less predictable. Do not exceed the recommended proportions of essential oil to carrier oil: 3-6 drops to 10 ml/2 tsp.

Oil	Code	Acne	Anxiety	Arthritis	Athlete's Foot	Blood pressure: High	Blood pressure: Low	Body odour	Bronchitis	Cellulite	Colds/chills	Constipation	Cystitis	Dandruff	Depression	Diarrhoea	Eczema	Fainting	Flatulence	Haemorrhoids	Hayfever	Headaches	Hormonal regulation	Indigestion	Influenza	Insomnia	Menopausal problems	Menstrual problems (general)	Irregular periods	Painful periods	Mental fatigue	Muscular aches	Nausea	Obesity	Pre-menstrual syndrome	Rheumatism	Sexual problems	Sinusitis	Stress	Throat infections	Travel sickness	Varicose veins	Warts	Water Retention
Basil	R, U		❀						❀		❀				❀			❀				❀		❀	❀			❀					❀		❀									
Bay	R			❀				❀	❀																											❀								
Benzoin	S			❀				❀	❀		❀		❀																															
Bergamot	R, U	❀	❀										❀		❀				❀																				❀					
Black Pepper	S			❀							❀	❀				❀			❀													❀	❀			❀								
Cedarwood	R	❀							❀					❀			❀								❀													❀						
Chamomile	R	❀	❀	❀										❀	❀	❀	❀					❀		❀		❀	❀	❀		❀			❀		❀	❀			❀					
Cinnamon	R							❀			❀					❀									❀								❀			❀		❀						
Comfrey	R				❀												❀											❀				❀												
Cypress	R		❀					❀			❀		❀							❀							❀	❀		❀		❀				❀						❀		❀
Eucalyptus	S	❀		❀					❀		❀		❀								❀	❀			❀			❀								❀		❀		❀				
Fennel	S											❀							❀					❀									❀	❀										
Frankincense	R										❀														❀											❀								
Geranium	R, U		❀								❀			❀									❀					❀							❀		❀							❀
Ginger	U										❀					❀			❀					❀								❀	❀			❀				❀	❀			
Grapefruit	U	❀																													❀			❀										❀
Hyssop	R, S					❀			❀															❀	❀																			
Jasmine	R	❀	❀												❀											❀											❀							
Juniper	R, U									❀	❀	❀	❀	❀	❀		❀			❀								❀				❀		❀		❀						❀		❀
Lavender	R, U	❀	❀	❀	❀	❀			❀		❀		❀	❀	❀		❀	❀				❀		❀	❀	❀		❀				❀	❀		❀	❀			❀	❀			❀	❀
Lemon	S	❀		❀					❀		❀		❀						❀					❀											❀					❀		❀		❀
Lemongrass	S		❀		❀			❀									❀					❀																		❀		❀		
Mandarin	U																		❀					❀																				
Marjoram	R		❀	❀					❀			❀										❀		❀								❀							❀					
Melissa	R, U		❀													❀					❀	❀	❀																❀					
Myrrh	S								❀		❀				❀		❀		❀																					❀				
Neroli	R		❀					❀							❀											❀	❀								❀		❀							
Nutmeg	S			❀							❀	❀							❀					❀									❀											
Orange	U		❀		❀										❀								❀	❀				❀																
Palmarosa	R	❀											❀																						❀									
Parsley	S			❀									❀																															❀
Patchouli	R	❀	❀		❀					❀				❀	❀	❀	❀																	❀			❀							
Peppermint	S							❀	❀		❀					❀			❀			❀		❀	❀							❀	❀			❀		❀				❀	❀	
Pine	S			❀					❀		❀		❀												❀						❀	❀				❀								❀
Rose	R		❀	❀											❀						❀					❀	❀	❀	❀	❀		❀			❀		❀		❀					
Rosemary	S				❀				❀		❀	❀			❀							❀		❀					❀		❀	❀				❀						❀		❀
Sage	S		❀	❀				❀	❀		❀	❀			❀							❀		❀				❀				❀				❀								❀
Clary Sage	R, S		❀		❀										❀				❀								❀	❀	❀	❀		❀			❀		❀		❀					
Sandalwood	R	❀	❀						❀		❀		❀		❀	❀			❀					❀				❀				❀	❀				❀			❀		❀		
Tea Tree	S				❀				❀		❀		❀												❀								❀										❀	
Thyme	S		❀						❀										❀					❀				❀				❀			❀	❀		❀						❀
Ylang Ylang	R		❀			❀									❀																		❀				❀							

CARRIER OILS

Vegetable carrier oils are more than just vehicles for essential oils, as they often have health-giving qualities of their own.
Choosing the appropriate carrier oil will add considerably to the dynamic nature of an aromatherapy massage and
can have specific benefits, such as helping to guard against heart disease or inflammatory diseases such as arthritis.

Vegetable oils are made up of essential fatty acids and contain the soluble vitamins A, D and E. Some vegetable oils also contain large amounts of gamma linoleic acid (GLA), used in the treatment of PMS. The fatty-acid compounds help to reduce blood cholesterol levels and strengthen cell membranes, thereby slowing down the formation of fine lines and wrinkles by helping the body to resist attack by free radicals.

Always use a cold-pressed, unrefined certified organic vegetable oil for the dilution of essential oils. The darker the colour and stronger the odour, the less refined the oil, so it will be rich in health-giving properties. Once the bottle is opened, keep it in the fridge.

Experiment with different types of carrier oil. Try adding a teaspoonful of a second vegetable oil to the base oil, as well as the essential oils, for a highly personal mixture. Remember that the weather affects the skin, and central heating and cold wind will cause it to dry out. These variations can be accommodated by changing the exotic vegetable oils used to enrich each blend.

Almond oil
A good source of vitamin D. It is suitable for all skin types, especially dry or irritated skin.

Avocado oil
This oil is easily absorbed into the deep tissues and is therefore excellent for mature skin. It can help to relieve the dryness and itching of psoriasis and eczema. Although it blends well with others, it has a distinctive fruity smell, so use it with essential oils with complementary fragrances.

Borage oil
One of the richest sources of GLA, it is useful for the relief of eczema and psoriasis, as well as for the symptoms of PMS.

Store carrier oils carefully to ensure their freshness.

Carrot oil
A valuable source of beta carotene, carrot oil is useful for healing scar tissue and soothing acne and irritated skin.

Evening primrose oil
A rich source of GLA, useful for the relief of eczema, psoriasis, dry skin, PMS and tender breasts. It is also suitable for face treatments, but as it is quite a sticky oil it should be mixed with a lighter oil, such as grapeseed, soya, peanut or peachnut, for this purpose.

Grapeseed oil
A non-greasy oil which suits most skin types. It is most readily available in a refined state, so it is best to mix it with almond oil to enrich the blend.

Hazelnut oil
Hazelnut oil has unusual astringent qualities that are valuable for oily and combination skins.

Jojoba oil
Because it is rich in vitamin E, jojoba oil is excellent for sensitive or oily complexions, but is also good for all skin types and penetrates more easily than other oils. It contains bactericidal properties, making it a useful oil for the treatment of acne.

Olive oil
Olive oil is too sticky for massage, but a good addition to a blend for mature or dry skin.

Peachnut oil
A fine oil rich in vitamin E and good for delicate skin. It encourages elasticity and suppleness, and is particularly suitable for face massage.

Peanut oil
Highly nutritious in its unrefined state, but this is rarely available. In its refined form it makes a good carrier oil for massage purposes, but it is helpful to enrich it with a more nutritious oil.

Safflower oil
This oil has a light texture and penetrates the skin well. It is cheap and readily available in an unrefined state, making it a useful base for a blend.

Sesame oil
When made from untoasted seeds, sesame oil is good for skin conditions. It has sun screening properties and is used in suncare preparations.

Sunflower oil
Sunflower is a light oil rich in vitamins and minerals. It can be enriched by adding more exotic oils.

Walnut oil
Contains small amounts of GLA, and has a pleasant, nutty aroma.

Wheat germ oil
Rich in vitamin E and useful for dry and mature skin. It is well known for its ability to heal scar tissue, smooth stretch marks and soothe burns. As it is too sticky to use on its own as a massage oil, add small amounts of it to a lighter oil, but do not use on people with wheat intolerance.

Carrier oils can be enriched with more exotic vegetable oils to create blends to suit specific skin types.

BLENDING AND STORING ESSENTIAL OILS

When essential oils are used for aromatherapy, different oils can be combined to increase their therapeutic effect.
As you become more practised in the art of blending you will begin to develop a nose for compatibility, in much the
same way as a perfumer blends scents, and you will be able to judge the best blend for your requirements by its aroma.
Once you have mixed your oils, store them carefully or use them immediately, as essential oils evaporate quickly.

Blending oils enables you to alleviate various physical and emotional symptoms in a single treatment, and while the combination of therapeutic properties is of prime importance, the value of fragrance should also be taken into account – no one enjoys taking unpleasant medicine, so don't underestimate the beneficial effects of a pleasing and sweet-smelling result when mixing your oils.

When blending oils for aromatherapy massage, the ratio of essential oil to carrier oil may vary, but as a general rule, up to 5 drops of essential oil in 10 ml/2 tsp carrier oil is enough for a body massage. This gives the recommended dilution for most massage purposes. However, if you are using oils for purely emotional problems, half the number of drops can be equally effective, while physical symptoms sometimes respond better to a higher percentage.

SYNERGY

When essential oils are blended, a chemical reaction occurs and the oils combine as a new compound. For example, when lavender is added to bergamot the sedative qualities of bergamot are increased; but if lemon is added to bergamot then its uplifting, refreshing aspect is enhanced. This process is known as synergy. Using this principle, oils can be blended so that they treat a person's emotional and physical needs at the same time. The blend can also be modified from treatment to treatment, depending on the time of day or the person's mood (for example, changing the balance of the blend, or substituting a different oil for one in the basic blend, can raise someone's spirits if they are low).

The natural aromas of essential oils blend as harmoniously as the plants from which they are distilled.

Be careful to mix enough of your chosen blend to complete a massage.

TOP, MIDDLE AND BASE NOTES

Essential oils are categorized by what are known as top, middle and base "notes". This is the way perfumers categorize scents, using different combinations of notes to create the balanced character of a new perfume. A good blend combines an oil from each category, and each oil is classified according to its dominant characteristic. You will eventually develop your own nose for which oils relate to each note. In general the fresh, herbaceous oils such as lemon, eucalyptus or tea tree are good top notes. The floral oils and some herb oils, such as lavender, geranium, chamomile and peppermint, make up the majority of the middle notes. The woody, resinous oils such as frankincense and sandalwood form the base notes. There are, however, some exceptions: rose and jasmine are unusually heady fragrances and although they are floral oils they are usually considered to be base notes.

Because they evaporate quickly, most blends should contain a higher percentage of top-note oil to each middle-note and base-note oil. For example, a well-balanced blend might be made up from 3 drops of orange (top note), 2 drops each of clary sage and geranium (both middle notes) and 2 drops of cedarwood (base note).

Top notes: fresh, light and immediately detectable because of their high evaporation rate.

Middle notes: the heart of the mixture, perceptible immediately after the top notes when smelling the blend for the first time.

Base notes: rich, heavy odours that linger and emerge fully only after more prolonged exposure to the blend.

It is easier to predict the synergistic effects of essential oils if not more than three are used in any one blend.

STORAGE OF ESSENTIAL OILS

Essential oils last for a relatively long time if a few simple precautions are taken. They should always be bought in dark-coloured glass bottles with a stopper that automatically dispenses them a drop at a time. Keep the lid firmly closed to prevent evaporation, and store them in a cool place out of direct sunlight and away from direct heat. The citrus oils tend to go off more quickly than other oils, so it is a good idea to buy them in small quantities as you need them. It is easy to tell if an oil has deteriorated: it will become cloudy and give off a distinctly unpleasant odour. Always keep all essential oils out of the reach of children.

Store blended oils in tightly stoppered bottles, away from bright light.

AROMATHERAPY BLENDS FOR EVERYDAY WELL-BEING

As you become familiar with the aromas and properties of essential oils, you will want to experiment with blends that especially suit you. One of the delights of aromatherapy is the blending together of oils for an enhanced therapeutic effect, making a new fragrance to soothe the senses at the same time.

Throughout this book you will find recipes for well-balanced blends designed to help with specific problems. However, the sense of smell is very individual, so if you find that you do not like a particular combination, try something else, always bearing in mind the actions of the oils and the recommended dilution rates. Let your nose tell you if a blend is harmonious, but above all if you enjoy its aroma.

Here are some suggestions to guide you to the oils that will help you recover from the strains of everyday life, or enhance your mood on happy occasions. Choose up to three of the suggested essential oils, mixing them with a carrier oil, to make your own blends.

A BLEND TO AID RELAXATION

Relaxation is particularly important following a stressful day at work. Choose up to three oils from this list: bergamot, German chamomile, clary sage, lavender, rosewood or sandalwood. To add an uplifting note, choose one of the other citrus oils, which will produce a blend that is relaxing and uplifting at the same time.

A BLEND TO DISPEL GLOOM

When everything seems grey, a blend of some of the invigorating oils could help turn the day around from one of gloom and despair to a more energetic one. Try a blend of up to three of the following oils to stimulate and cleanse the system and make you feel more lively: black pepper, cypress, eucalyptus, fennel, ginger, grapefruit, jasmine, juniper, lemon, nutmeg, peppermint, rosemary or tea tree.

Enjoy the therapeutic effects of essential oils every day by adding them to beauty and bath preparations.

An aromatherapy massage is an ideal way to relieve tension or stimulate a sluggish system.

A BLEND FOR STIFF MUSCLES

Everyone can suffer from minor muscular aches and pains from time to time. They may be brought on by unusual physical exercise – from gardening or dancing to sporting activities – or simply by sitting or standing too long in an uncomfortable position. At such times the warming oils that bring blood back into the aching muscles are the most helpful. Choose from the following list: benzoin, black pepper, clary sage, eucalyptus, ginger, grapefruit, jasmine, juniper, lavender, lemon, marjoram, nutmeg, orange, peppermint or rosemary.

A REMEDY TO SOOTHE THE SKIN AFTER SUNBATHING

Prolonged sunbathing, particularly in the middle and hottest part of the day, can have a devastating effect on the skin. It encourages premature ageing and can be very painful. Prevention is, of course, better than cure, but if you are feeling tender and providing the skin is not actually burnt and broken, a gentle massage with a soothing oil is very comforting and moisturizing. Use rose and chamomile essential oils, and include some wheat germ oil in the blend which will also help to heal the skin.

A REMEDY FOR OVER-INDULGENCE

If you have had too much to drink, try to drink several glasses of water before sleeping, to help alleviate the dehydration caused by an excess of alcohol. Drink plenty of water and orange juice at breakfast to help speed up detoxification and, if you can, eat some wholemeal toast with a yeast spread. A blend of up to three of the following oils may help restore your system to normal good health after eating or drinking too much: black pepper, fennel, geranium, ginger, juniper, orange, peppermint.

The warm fragrance of essential oil of rose is an ideal choice for raising the spirits and restoring a sense of well-being.

ESSENTIAL OILS FOR TRAVELLERS

If travelling is a source of anxiety for you, or if you suffer from travel sickness, essential oils can help to calm both the mind and the stomach. The simplest way to use them when you are travelling is to put a couple of drops on to a tissue or handkerchief and smell them frequently during the journey. Useful oils for this purpose are peppermint, mandarin or neroli.

A BLEND FOR RAISING THE SPIRITS

For the days when the ordinary activities of life seem too difficult, there are a number of oils that can help raise the spirits: benzoin, bergamot, cedarwood, clary sage, frankincense, geranium, grapefruit, jasmine, mandarin, nutmeg, orange, rose, rosewood or ylang ylang. A blend of up to three essential oils from this list can give you back your usual zest for life.

A BLEND TO BRING WARMTH AND COMFORT

After struggling with bitter winds and the cold of winter, there are some warming and comforting essential oils that can be very nourishing when you are feeling emotionally, as well as physically, cold. Blend benzoin, ginger, orange and rosewood together and allow them to envelop you in their special aroma.

An aphrodisiac blend

In a long-term relationship the intimate physical bond between partners may weaken or cease to exist. A long illness, overwork or emotional crises can also contribute to a lack of sexual interest. At such times the non-sexual but loving touch of massage can play an important part in rediscovering the sexual intimacy that has been missing. Essential oils that may help are: black pepper, cedarwood, clary sage, fennel, frankincense, ginger, jasmine, rose and sandalwood. Bear in mind that this is an area where it is especially important to take into account both partners' personal preferences for fragrance.

A nuptial blend

There is only one blend to choose before a wedding: jasmine and rose, respectively the king and queen of fragrances, and neroli, to calm the nerves. This luxurious blend will bring the essence of calm to the beginning of married life.

A blend to instil peacefulness

Frankincense, sandalwood, neroli and ylang ylang blend together to create a rich perfume of peace. This blend can help recreate feelings of tranquillity and reduce feelings of fragmentation. It can be valuable in helping to reconnect you to your strong inner core and regain peace in your life.

Blending essential oils

Before you begin, wash and dry your hands and make sure that all your utensils are clean and dry. Have your essential oils at the ready, but leave the lids on the bottles until they are required.

1 Carefully measure out 10 ml/2 tsp of your chosen vegetable oil.

2 Gently pour the measured vegetable oil into your blending bowl.

3 Add the first essential oil a drop at a time. Add the remaining oils a drop at a time, up to a maximum of 6 drops, and mix gently with a clean, dry cocktail stick or toothpick, to blend. Rub a little of the blend in your hands to test the fragrance.

SING ESSENTIAL OILS

You can soak and splash in them, feed your skin, sensually smooth them all over, or simply breathe in their wonderful aromas. The pleasure and versatility of aromatic oils make them one of nature's kindest gifts. Essential oils contain the active ingredients of a plant in a highly concentrated and potent form. They therefore need to be treated with care and should never be applied directly to the skin undiluted. Massage, aromatic baths and inhalations are some of the most effective ways to use essential oils therapeutically, and are described on the following pages.

There are many ways of surrounding yourself with the uplifting or relaxing fragrances of the oils. Apart from vaporizers and sprays for scenting your home, you can experiment with your own blends of scents to create luxurious body oils, lotions and treatments for your hair. Wooden balls scented with aromatic oils will add fragrance to drawers used for storing clothes. Alternatively, you can scent paper drawer-liners and padded coat hangers with a few drops of essential oils such as melissa or bergamot, or cedarwood to deter moths. You can even deodorize your shoes with a drop of parsley or pine oil. Away from home, the most portable way of using essential oils is to sprinkle 3–4 drops on to a handkerchief and inhale the fragrance.

Add a few drops of an essential oil to hot water
to enjoy its unique aroma.

OILS IN THE AIR

A lingering smell, whether pleasant or not, is usually the first thing you notice when you enter a room, and it can strongly affect the way you feel. Fragrancing the home to delight the senses is an old tradition. For centuries the Chinese have suspended balls of jasmine flowers over the bed to clear the air and promote pleasant dreams, while bowls of potpourri, scented sachets and pomanders have a long history. Today, the methods of scenting a room are many and diverse. They can help prevent ill-health, balance the emotions and disguise unpleasant smells such as cigarette smoke or stale cooking odours.

LIVING ROOMS

Rose, geranium, orange and lavender are pleasing and uplifting scents for a room, used individually or blended together.

For an exotic, intimate atmosphere, use sandalwood or patchouli, or to unwind in the evening try geranium, lavender, sandalwood or ylang ylang.

Perfumes for parties

Clary sage or jasmine will create a heady, "feel-good" atmosphere for a party, or use orange, lemongrass or neroli for a lighter, fresher touch.

For a festive blend, choose from the spicier oils such as frankincense, cedarwood, sandalwood, cinnamon and orange.

STUDIES AND OFFICES

Useful oils for the workplace are basil, rosemary, bergamot, lemon and melissa. Bergamot and lemon are particularly antiseptic, and lemon has the added advantage of helping efficiency. Basil stimulates a tired brain and rosemary is a great aid to concentration. Rosemary is also helpful in relieving headaches. If you are feeling overwrought try clary sage or juniper, but watch the dosage as too much will cause sleepiness.

If you work in a large, open-plan space, fragrancing the whole area may not be a viable option. Sprinkle a few drops on a handkerchief or add a few drops of oil to a cup of hot water on your desk.

BEDROOMS

Whether to ensure a restful night's sleep or to turn your bedroom into a place of passion, fragrancing the bedroom just before bedtime will create an appropriate atmosphere. Rose, neroli and lavender are delightful all-purpose oils for the bedroom. Perfume your pillow with 2–3 drops of a relaxing oil to help you unwind, or one for insomnia if you have sleep problems. For a different mood, try an aphrodisiac like ylang ylang or be extravagant and use rose or jasmine, the two most luxurious and expensive essential oils.

Use lavender to freshen a musty spare room to make it welcoming for guests. Clear the atmosphere of a sick room with bergamot, eucalyptus or juniper.

KITCHENS AND BATHROOMS

Use tea tree, eucalyptus, melissa, lemongrass or the closely related citronella in a diffuser to keep insects at bay. Pine, lemon or tea tree can be used on a damp cloth to disinfect surfaces.

Vaporized molecules of any essential oil will neutralize airborne bacteria, but some – such as tea tree, bergamot, lemon, pine and lavender – are particularly antiseptic. Use these in a diffuser or room spray.

When you buy scented candles, make sure they have been made using natural essential oils.

DIFFUSING FRAGRANCES

Vaporizers come in many forms, but all work on the same principle. The reservoir is filled with water, to which are added drops of essential oil. The reservoir is then heated, causing the water to evaporate and the warm oil to release its perfume.

Make sure there is a suitable distance between the source of the heat and the reservoir for oil and water. This will reduce the risk of completely evaporating the water and thus burning the oil. The vaporizer should also be easy to clean ready for use with a different oil.

The simplest type of vaporizer has a candle as the heat source; a more efficient, but more expensive, type is the electric vaporizer, which is useful when you want to disperse oils for a long period of time without the necessity of frequent supervision. Some electric vaporizers have a silent fan that disperses the evaporating oils; others employ a heated ceramic dish. Either would be suitable for a child's or invalid's bedroom.

Simple vaporizers for essential oils disperse the fragrance quickly and effectively, and also make attractive ornaments.

Add a few drops of essential oil to an oil lamp to scent a room.

How to use a vaporizer

Whenever you use a vaporizer of any kind, do make certain that you place it in a safe position, out of the reach of children and pets.

The number of drops of oil used in a burner depends on the size of the room: 2–3 drops for a small room, and as many as 6–10 for a larger one. It is better to use fewer drops and refresh the burner more frequently, rather than use too many and saturate the room with scent. Remember that your sensitivity to the scent will decrease, but this does not mean that the aroma is not still present and probably still quite strong.

Room sprays

To make a room spray, blend 10 drops of essential oil in 105 ml/7 tbsp water. 15 ml/1 tbsp vodka or pure alcohol added to the solution will act as a preservative, but this is optional. Shake well before filling a sprayer.

Humidifiers

You can add your favourite oil to the water of a humidifier or improvise by adding 5 drops of essential oil to a small bowl of water placed on top of a radiator.

Ring burners

Use the heat from light bulbs to release perfumed oils. Small ring burners, usually made of porcelain or aluminium, sit over the top of the bulb. Add a few drops of essential oil, and the heat from the bulb will gently vaporize the oil.

Wood fires

Sprinkle drops of cypress, cedarwood, pine or sandalwood over the logs to be used about an hour before lighting the fire and then burn them to release your favourite aroma.

Scented candles

Wax candles can be bought ready-impregnated with essential oils and are a delightful way of fragrancing a room. Or you can add a few drops of essential oil to an oil lamp for the same effect.

Potpourri

Add a few drops of an appropriate flowery or spicy essential oil to refresh tired potpourri.

To make a simmering potpourri, place a mixture of scented flowers and leaves (without any fixatives or additives) in a bowl of water and heat gently from below – a candle flame may well be sufficient. The aroma is not long-lasting, but is much stronger than that of dry potpourri. Add about 1 cupful of dried plant material to 1 litre/ 1¾ pints of water.

For a sleep-enhancing simmering potpourri, blend ½ cup lime flowers, ¼ cup chamomile flowers, 15 ml/1 tbsp sweet marjoram and 15 ml/ 1 tbsp lavender flowers. For a more refreshing, uplifting blend, try ½ cup lemon verbena leaves, ¼ cup jasmine flowers, 30 ml/2 tbsp lemon peel and 5 ml/1 tsp coriander seeds.

QUICK THERAPIES WITH ESSENTIAL OILS

In the middle of a busy day you may not have the time for a leisurely, relaxing bath or a full-body massage, but you can still benefit from the therapeutic effects of essential oils using these simple methods. The heat of the water will release the aromas of the oils immediately, so have everything ready for the treatment before you add them.

STEAM INHALATIONS

For problems like colds and sinus congestion, a steam inhalation warms and moistens the membranes, and the use of essential oils helps to open and relax the airways. Just boil a kettle, pour approximately ½ litre/1 pint hot water into a bowl, add the oils and inhale deeply. Use up to 5 drops for a strong medicinal effect, in cases of colds or chestiness, or just 2 drops for a gentler relaxing effect on the air passages.

RECOMMENDED ESSENTIAL OILS

A blend for nasal congestion:
For a stuffed-up feeling, maybe combined with tiredness, use 3 drops eucalyptus and 2 drops peppermint.

To ease a tight, tense chest:
For tension causing poor breathing, relax the airways with 4 drops lavender and 3 drops frankincense.

CAUTION: Do not overdo an inhalation, and if you have high blood pressure or asthma, seek medical advice before using steam.

For respiratory complaints in particular, steam inhalations are very helpful.

COMPRESSES

Hot or cold compresses are excellent ways to use oils for problems such as sprains and muscular aches. Cold compresses are suitable for use on acute injuries such as a strain or sprain, with swelling or bruising, though you should of course always seek medical advice in cases of serious injury. To make a cold compress, pour cold water over some ice in a bowl, add essential oils and soak a pad in the water before placing over the affected area and binding firmly in place.

For older injuries, with no swelling or inflammation, for chronic muscle pain and for arthritic or rheumatic pain, a hot compress may be more useful. For a hot compress: have the water as hot as you can comfortably bear. Pour it into a bowl, add the oils and use as above. Use 3–4 drops of essential oil in 250 ml/8 fl oz hot water (enough to fill an average-sized cereal bowl).

Hand and footbaths are a simple way of enjoying the benefits of essential oils.

RECOMMENDED ESSENTIAL OILS

A first aid remedy:
The ideal essential oil for a cold compress
is lavender, and this can be very useful
in many first aid situations.
Use 4 drops to a bowl of
iced water. Keep the pad on firmly
for at least 20 minutes, preferably
with the affected limb raised if there is
any swelling.

A blend for muscular pain:
For muscular aches and pains,
try using 2 drops each of rosemary and
marjoram in a bowl of hot water.
Apply the compress for
30 minutes.

HAND AND FOOTBATHS

A quick way to use essential oils is to make a hand or footbath; two-thirds fill a large bowl with hot water and add 3–4 drops of oils. The warmth of the water itself helps the blood vessels to dilate, and this can be very helpful in treating conditions such as tension headaches and migraines, when the blood vessels in the head are frequently engorged with blood. Try a foot or handbath at an early stage of a headache and see if you can drain away the excess stress.

RECOMMENDED ESSENTIAL OILS

A blend to improve circulation:
For poor circulation and cold extremities, use
2 drops lavender and 2 drops marjoram oils.

Blends for aching muscles:
For tension and stiffness:
If stiffness is due to over-exertion, try a blend
of 2 drops rosemary and 2 drops pine.
To refresh hot, aching feet or hands:
Use a mixture of 2 drops peppermint and
2 drops lemon.

A footbath will not only relieve aching feet, but warm and invigorate the whole body.

THE AROMATIC BATH

A bath with essential oils is one of the simplest and most effective aromatherapy treatments. It can be stimulating or relaxing, depending on the temperature of the water and whether you choose oils with uplifting or calming properties. In the bath, the therapeutic action of the oils is twofold: they are absorbed through the skin, moisturizing the dermis and entering the circulatory system, and at the same time their aromas are inhaled, stimulating the brain and increasing your sense of well-being. An aromatic bath can detoxify the body and help with problems like cellulite, joint stiffness, general aches and pains, colds and headaches. It will also tone and condition the skin and relieve anxiety and tension.

RUNNING THE BATH

Bath temperature and the time spent in the tub are important. A cooler bath is more stimulating and warmer water relaxes. Very hot water is damaging, however: it causes blood vessels and capillaries to expand and increases the heart rate. You should particularly avoid hot water if you have varicose veins, haemorrhoids, high blood pressure or are pregnant. A 15–20 minute soak is long enough before skin cells over-hydrate, or swell with water.

Use aromatherapy treatments to enhance your bathtime routine.

RECOMMENDED ESSENTIAL OILS

For stimulation:
Bergamot, cypress, eucalyptus, fennel, geranium, juniper, lavender, lemon, lemongrass, peppermint, pine, rosemary, thyme.

For relaxation:
Basil, cedarwood, chamomile, frankincense, hyssop, juniper, lavender, marjoram, melissa, neroli, patchouli, rose, sage, sandalwood, ylang ylang.

A morning blend:
For a refreshing, uplifting bath, try a blend of 3 drops bergamot and 2 drops geranium.

An evening blend:
To relax and unwind after a long day, make a blend of 3 drops lavender and 2 drops ylang ylang to add to your bath.

Bath oil formula (for three baths):
Mix a bath oil with a combination of up to three essential oils, up to 5 drops of each, in 15 ml/1 tbsp skin softening base oil. Choose oils with complementary effects. Use a third of the mixture for each bath.

OILS FOR THE BATH

Essential oils are the best way of making a bath both aromatic and therapeutic. They sink into the skin easily and at the same time impart their lovely herbal or floral fragrances.

You can add 5 drops of essential oil directly to the bath: they will float on the surface in a fine film and evaporate, giving you the full benefit of their aroma instantly.

If you want to absorb them more through the skin you can disperse them through the water by mixing with a base carrier oil such as sweet almond, apricot kernel, jojoba or evening primrose (these rich base oils all nourish and rejuvenate the skin in their own right, leaving it smooth and well moisturized).

THE STIMULATING BATH

The stimulating oils are best for the morning to get you started or to revive you at the end of a busy day before an evening out.

Keep the water fairly cool and use an invigorating bath mitt to rub down, enlivening the skin and stimulating the circulation. When you've soaked, rinse yourself with water as cold as you can bear, either by splashing directly from the tap or shower, or by adding more cold water to cool down your bath.

As you get out of the bath, either slap yourself dry to make the skin tingle or rub yourself vigorously with a towel.

THE RELAXING BATH

To calm yourself after a fraught day or to prepare yourself for a peaceful night's sleep, turn your bathroom into a private sanctuary. First, choose a time when you won't be interrupted by family or telephone calls. Keep the light in the room soft if possible, or use an eye mask or burn aromatic candles. Plants not only look good in the bathroom but also create an oxygenated atmosphere. Support your head with a bath pillow, close your eyes and inhale deeply. Concentrate on your breathing, empty your mind and let the oils soothe away the stresses and strains of the day. After a 15–20 minute soak, get out slowly and wrap yourself in a large, warm towel.

THE THERAPEUTIC BATH

Adding essential oils to a warm bath is also an effective way to exploit their physiological healing properties, particularly for skin problems as the warmth of the water will soften and relax the skin, allowing the oils to be absorbed readily.

RECOMMENDED ESSENTIAL OILS

For dermatitis:
Chamomile, hyssop, lavender.

For eczema:
Chamomile, geranium, hyssop, juniper, rosemary, myrrh.

For psoriasis:
Bergamot, chamomile, lavender.

For arthritis/rheumatism:
Chamomile, eucalyptus, juniper, lavender, rosemary, thyme.

A blend for aching muscles:
Add 3 drops marjoram and 2 drops chamomile essential oils to the bath.

SHOWERS AND COLD RINSES

Invigorating jets of water are ideal for getting the blood pumping and there's no need to forego the benefits of aromatic oils. Skin tends to be sluggish in the cold winter months but sloughing off dead top layers can help regenerate cells and allow moisturizers to be absorbed more easily. Showers are ideal for smoothing skin with exfoliating rubs using wet salt, a loofah or a friction mitt. Soften loofahs and mitts first in warm water. Soft bristle brushes can also help to get the circulation going with gentle massage on problem areas like hips and thighs. To keep brushes and mitts fresh, always rinse them and hang them up to dry.

Essential oils can be used under the shower: mix a base oil with invigorating essences, pour on to a clean face-cloth or sponge and rub all over the body in a circular motion while showering. A cold shower after cleansing improves the circulation and tightens skin pores.

Start off your shower or bath routine by whisking off dead skin cells with a friction mitt. Moisten it with warm water or softening oils such as sweet almond or evening primrose. Concentrate on outer thighs, working from the knee in upward circular movements across the buttocks.

Wait until the bath is almost full before adding the oils, as they evaporate quickly.

AFTER-BATH BODY TREATMENTS

Moisturizing oils and lotions applied after the bath or shower help to nourish the skin, keeping it soft and supple.
As you get older your skin dehydrates since the oil glands do not produce as much oil as in youth. Apply a body oil all over,
starting from the feet and working right up to the neck and tips of the ears. Avoid talcum powders which clog the pores
and tend to have a drying effect.

PROBLEM ZONES

Pay special attention to your hands, feet and elbows and spend some time each week looking after them.

Hands and nails

Hands and nails take some rough treatment with everyday chores. The ideal time for a manicure or pedicure is after soaking in a bath, when nails and skin have been softened by the water, making it easy to clean around the nail bed and to clip uneven nails without snagging.

Fragile or flaky nails benefit from a rich, nourishing treatment: rub them with apricot kernel, wheat germ or jojoba oil.

Condition hands and nails with a simple finger-pulling exercise. Spread and stretch the fingers straight out; massage each finger with oil, working from the tip of the nails to the cuticles and up to each knuckle.

RECOMMENDED ESSENTIAL OILS

To soothe and moisturize your hands:
Blend 5 drops each patchouli, lavender and lemon essential oils with
15 ml/1 tbsp sweet almond oil.

For a deodorizing and soothing footbath:
Blend 3 drops each cypress and lavender in a bowl of warm water.

For chilblains:
Blend 3 drops geranium and 1 drop each lavender and rosemary in 15 ml/1 tbsp sweet almond oil.

Body oil formula:
For a lasting effect, mix up to three essential oils, 5 drops of each in 30 ml/2 tbsp base oil. If you want to make up a larger quantity of body oil, use a concentration of 3% essential oil in the base oil.

Feet

Feet are often neglected until they hurt. Polish hard skin with a handful of damp salt or use a pumice stone. While in the bath, bend one knee, grip the toes and then work with the fingers, massaging in an upward direction from the toes to the heels and up the calves in order to stimulate blood flow and relax tired feet. Massage a body oil into the feet after a bath, shower or pedicure.

Soften the feet after a bath by massaging with a body oil to which you have added essential oils. Work between the toes and then around the tougher skin and heel areas. Finish with sweeping movements all over to stimulate the circulation.

Apply body oil to the arms with smooth upward strokes, concentrating on the elbows and upper arms where the skin is often rougher and drier.

Elbows

Elbows can soon build up hard protective layers of grey, unsightly skin. A good softener for tough elbows is a sweet almond oil and oatmeal scrub. Mix 45 ml/3 tbsp sweet almond oil with 45 ml/ 3 tbsp fine oatmeal and mix to a paste with fresh milk or yogurt. Smooth and rub over the elbows and any grey, goosey areas of skin around the upper arms. Add 6 drops of fennel essential oil if arms are flabby.

Another great booster for rough elbows is the traditional remedy of cutting a lemon in half, squeezing out the juice and rubbing the elbows in the hollow of the lemon.

When it comes to applying body oil, the back, neck and shoulders are often neglected because they are difficult to reach, but these are key areas for releasing tension and the skin needs to be nourished, so smooth as far as possible, or enlist the help of a friend.

BEAUTY BASICS

Looking good starts with great skin, and aromatherapy can help you achieve this in various ways: the remarkable penetrative properties of essential oils make them excellent moisturizers, and the wide range of their properties means there is always the right oil for any condition. For instance, rosemary stimulates the circulation and thyme helps the cells to regenerate. As well as being stimulating to the lymphatic system, which helps cleanse the tissue that causes sluggish skin, essential oils can be used as part of your daily skincare routine and to treat specific problems such as acne.

FEED YOUR SKIN

Skin needs to be fed and nourished – inside and out. Healthy diets can keep the body in shape but to keep skin in peak condition it needs to have a ready supply of valuable vitamins and minerals. Many factors can drain the body of this valuable resource – too much over-processed food, caffeine, alcohol, nicotine, sunlight, central heating, carbon monoxide and habitual drug-taking. The effects of these can build up and attack the skin, so from time to time you need to give it a break.

A one-day fruit and vegetable diet is an excellent regime to adopt once a month to cleanse your body and give a boost to your system.

RECOMMENDED ESSENTIAL OILS

For dry skin:
Chamomile, geranium, lavender, hyssop, rose, patchouli, sandalwood, ylang ylang.

For sensitive skin:
Chamomile, lavender, neroli, rose, sandalwood.

For oily skin:
Bergamot, cedarwood, cypress, fennel, lavender, lemon, geranium, juniper, frankincense, sage.

Blends for a facial steam:
Add 5 drops chamomile to a large bowl of hot water for a soothing steam or try lavender, peppermint, thyme or rosemary to stimulate, or comfrey or fennel for their healing properties. Put a towel over your head and lower your face over the steam for 5 minutes.

Nourishing blends for any skin type:
To a 25 g/1 oz pot of unperfumed skin cream, add either 3 drops rose and 3 drops sandalwood, or 4 drops neroli and 2 drops rose.

THE EFFECTS OF STRESS

If you become stressed, the small muscles close to the skin tend to contract. This can leave your skin under-nourished with blood, and over time your complexion and skin tone suffer. Apart from dealing with underlying worries, the skin itself can also be helped with essential oils.

SKIN TYPES

Choose the right oils for your skin type and use them to blend your own cleansers, toners, masks and moisturizers. Remember that skin types can vary: skin may be drier in winter or more prone to oiliness around the time of your period, and it can change as you get older. So review the oils you use to suit your skin now and vary them to meet the changing needs of your complexion.

Combination skin has an oily T-zone from the forehead down to the nose and chin area, and may be normal or dry elsewhere. If you have a complexion like this, double up on the treatments, using oils for oily skin on the greasy patches.

CLEANSERS

Choose the correct essential oils for your skin type and blend them with an ordinary unperfumed brand of cleanser, liquid soap or tissue-off lotion or cream, and they will do nature's work of rebalancing the skin.

Pay particular attention to oily areas of the face when cleansing the skin.

For a deep-cleansing facial steam, boil some water, cool slightly and add 5 drops of essential oil. Put a towel over your head and steam your face for 5 minutes.

TONERS

Essential oils are the gentlest way of toning up. Rose-water for normal or dry/sensitive skin, or witch-hazel for oilier skin, are ideal toners. Or you can blend your own flower waters: simply take a sterile, 100 ml/3½ fl oz bottle of dark-coloured glass, fill it with spring water and add 30 drops of your chosen essential oils. Leave in a cool, dark place for a few days, then filter the water through a coffee filter-paper into a second, similar bottle. Keep it in the fridge.

Herbal infusions also make ideal toners. Boil a cup of water and infuse chamomile, marigold, rosehip or nettle teas. Add 2 drops of orange or lavender oil to the infusion and leave to cool. Oily skin benefits from juniper or lemongrass essential oils, whereas drier skins would appreciate rose or sandalwood.

FACIAL OILS AND CREAMS

Well-moisturized skin is soft and supple, reflects a healthy glow and ages less quickly. Younger skin needs only light conditioning, whereas older skin needs specific nourishing treatments. Most moisturizers soothe and sit on the surface of the skin, but essential oils, with their fine molecular structure, work their way through from the surface to the inner dermis (the skin's deeper regenerating layer). Mixed with the correct amount of base oil, pure essential oils do not clog up the pores: they are light enough to be absorbed spontaneously by the skin.

Use 30 ml/2 tbsp base oil and add 6 drops of essential oils (use a maximum of three different oils) to suit your skin's individual needs. Alternatively, add 6 drops of essential oils to a 25 g/ 1 oz pot of your favourite skin cream.

As with all essential oils blends, it is best if you mix up only small amounts of cream and oil at a time to avoid deterioration.

FACE MASKS

Both clay and oatmeal are ideal ingredients for a face mask. Fuller's earth is a natural powdered clay which can be mixed into a paste with hot water. Cool and then add yogurt for a smoother consistency. Similarly, finely ground oatmeal can be mixed into a paste and left to cool. Add 2 drops of essential oils to suit your skin type per 5 ml/1 tsp of paste. Smooth on to your face, leave to dry slightly and then sponge off. For particularly dry sensitive skin, add 5 ml/1 tbsp evening primrose oil to give a more moisturizing mask. When applying, avoid the eye area.

Eye treats

While relaxing with a face mask on, close the eyes and cover them with cotton pads soaked in rose-water, or soothe with two slices of cucumber.

Use essential oils to make delicately-scented flower waters to tone your skin.

RECOMMENDED ESSENTIAL OILS

A remedy for odd spots:
If you are prone to occasional spots, mix 1 drop of neroli, lemon and lavender in 5 ml/1 tsp base oil and treat just the affected area. For a single spot, use a cotton bud and dab on one spot of undiluted sandalwood.

ACNE

Because of their bactericidal, anti-inflammatory and rebalancing properties, essential oils are ideal skin treatments for acne sufferers.

It is a mistake to scrub oily skin over-zealously: this only activates the sebaceous glands which in turn produce more sebum. If you suffer from pustular acne, avoid excessive facial steams which may spread the condition to other areas of the face: use a mask instead.

From day to day, use a cleanser and moisturizer formulation suitable for sensitive skin, adding 2 drops of juniper, which is stimulating and anti-septic. Opt for a deeper clay-type mask treatment once a week, adding 2 drops of juniper to heal, soothe and tighten the skin, or eucalyptus which is anti-inflammatory, antiseptic and antibiotic. Increase your dietary intake of vitamin E, which is a great skin healer.

COLD SORES

Cold sores are small blisters on the lips or surrounding area which are caused by the virus *Herpes simplex*. It normally lies dormant in nerve cells but can surface when resistance is lowered, such as following a simple cold or 'flu. Any lip sore that persists should be treated medically, but for the common cold sore a dab of undiluted tea tree oil will help.

BROKEN VEINS

These small, red, spider-like thread veins often appear on the surface of the skin around the cheek area. They are broken capillaries and seem to affect those with a delicate or fragile skin type. Hot and cold elements, along with stimulants such as alcohol or caffeine, can trigger this condition. To treat it at home the secret is to protect the skin from losing excess moisture and to give it extra essential oil treatments using parsley, geranium, chamomile, rosemary or cypress in a heavy base oil.

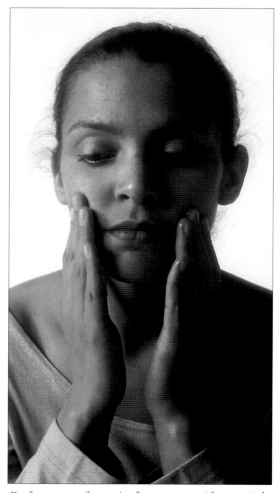

Perfume your favourite face cream with essential oils appropriate to your skin type.

FACIAL MASSAGE

Giving your face a regular massage helps the skin to absorb oils and creams more easily. Give skin a clear start with our step-by-step facial, using a blend of essential oils suited to your skin type in a nourishing carrier oil. This simple routine will tone your skin, helping it to retain its youthful elasticity and smoothing out any fine lines. It will also improve your circulation, speeding up the elimination of toxins from the tissues and giving your face a healthy glow.

1 Pour a little oil into your hand and apply all over the face, avoiding the eyes.

2 With the backs of your hands, gently tap the skin around the jaw line and underneath the chin.

3 Apply small circular movements to the chin area, using your thumbs, to tone, help circulation and eliminate toxins.

4 Make an "oooh"-shape mouth. Massage the skin on either side of your mouth with your fingertips, easing out fine lines.

5 With your fingertips, press along the top of the cheekbones and massage outward up to the temples to release toxins.

6 Press above the bridge of the nose and under the eyebrows. Hold for 5 seconds, then smooth across the eyebrows and up to the temples.

7 To relieve tension, apply firm pressure with the fingertips at either side of the temples and rotate backward.

8 Finally, stroke up the forehead from the brow to the hairline with the palm of the hands, smoothing out fine lines.

HEALTHY HAIR

Hair can define your image and style but it is also a mirror of your health. Emotional or physical problems can soon result in a lack of bounce and shine. As with your skin, keeping hair in peak condition is a combination of caring for it on the surface and nurturing it from inside with a well-balanced diet.

HAIR TYPES

How you treat your hair depends largely on its type. Make sure you use the most appropriate treatment for your kind of hair.

Dry hair

Dry hair is rough to touch, thick in texture and dries out at the first sign of heated rollers or tongs. Avoid chemical colorants and perms and opt for shampoos and conditioners containing jojoba and almond oils. Hot-oil treatments allow essential oils to soak in easily and condition the hair. After massaging warm oil into the scalp, wrap the head in a warm towel and leave on for half an hour.

Normal hair

Normal hair is glossy with plenty of natural body and bounce. An occasional hot-oil scalp treatment will keep it looking good and growing healthily.

Greasy hair

Greasy hair tends to look dull, lank, lacks body and won't hold a style. Central heating and environmental elements aggravate the condition, but it can stem from a hormonal imbalance. Check your diet and avoid harsh degreasing shampoos. Clean brushes and combs weekly. Plastic brushes are better for brushing through as bristle continually stimulates the scalp. Choose light conditioning rinses to detangle but try a scalp massage to regulate the oil-producing sebaceous glands.

Combination hair

If the ends of your hair are dry or normal but it is greasy at the roots, avoid using hot appliances near the scalp and keep the ends regularly trimmed. Use a scalp treatment with oils for greasy hair but don't comb through to the ends.

RECOMMENDED ESSENTIAL OILS

For dry hair:
Rose, sandalwood, ylang ylang, lavender, geranium.

For normal hair:
Geranium, lavender, lemongrass, rosemary.

For greasy hair:
Basil, eucalyptus, cedarwood, chamomile, lemongrass, cypress, sage, rosemary.

Scalp massage oil formula:
For the base oil, choose from sweet almond, apricot kernel, avocado, jojoba, evening primrose or sunflower.
Choose up to three essential oils and use 5 drops of each in 30 ml/2 tbsp base oil. Warm the oils by placing the container in a bowl of boiling water, then massage into the scalp. Wrap with a hot towel, leave for 15 minutes and then shampoo.

HAIR PROBLEMS

Apart from improving the condition of your hair generally, essential oils can help with specific scalp problems.

Dandruff

There are two types: dry and the more common oily. It's not catching! It can be caused by factors such as chemical body changes, stress, poor eating habits or incorrect application of hair products. Both flaky and dry scalps can be treated with essential oils. Use special dandruff shampoos and conditioning rinses and treat the scalp by gently massaging with suitable oils. For a flaky scalp use patchouli and tea tree. For a dry, itchy scalp, try cedarwood and lavender.

Grey hair

Grey hair is more porous and needs extra conditioning, particularly if it is chemically treated or coloured. Use a blend suitable for dry hair, adding essential oil enhancers like chamomile to lighten or sage to darken any discoloration.

Hair loss

Hair coming out in handfuls is often due to a hormonal imbalance, stress or anxiety, so the first step is to learn to relax. Any unusual thinning patch should be looked at by a trichologist but, as a general remedy, massage the scalp using a blend containing lavender and rosemary oils.

A few drops of geranium oil on a hairbrush add a delightful fragrance to the hair, while chamomile makes an excellent rinse for fair hair.

SCALP MASSAGE

This is a wonderful way to condition hair, stimulate the scalp and relieve tension. You can use these steps to treat your own hair, but it's even more relaxing if you can persuade a friend to help, especially if your hair is long.

1 Shampoo the hair and towel dry. Comb through with a wide-tooth comb. Tilt your head back and pour some blended oil on to the hairline, massaging in with thumbs on the temples and fingers spread apart over the centre of the head.

4 Work from front to back, following the natural flow of blood, from the forehead, frontal hairline, temples and sides, over the crown of the head to the base of the neck. If the scalp feels particularly tight, concentrate on areas where it doesn't want to move. At the base of the skull, press firmly and push the whole scalp up toward the crown to release tension.

2 Loosely run fingers and oil over the top of the scalp from front to back, lifting hair at the crown. Keep dipping your fingertips in the oil as you begin the massage so that there is enough on the hair to spread right through to the ends.

3 Massage the head with kneading movements. Grip and push against the scalp, which should gently rotate against the skull. Concentrate on one area at a time, with the hands positioned on either side of the scalp.

5 Pull any extra oil through the hair, working out from the roots to the ends. Make sure all the hair is well oiled, then wrap it in a towel and leave for at least 15 minutes before shampooing.

AROMATHERAPY MASSAGE

An aromatherapy massage is a wonderful way to unwind and ease stored tensions, triggering the body's natural healing processes by stimulating the flow of blood and lymph fluid. At the same time, the aromas are acting upon the emotional centre in the brain (the limbic system) which governs the way you feel.

CHOOSING ESSENTIAL OILS FOR MASSAGE

Aromatherapists never start a massage immediately. In order to provide the most effective treatment, the therapist needs to ascertain the state of mind and body of the individual, and establish whether there are any specific problems to attend to. Is the problem physical? Is it mental? Is it a combination of both? To help them to treat a wide variety of complaints, aromatherapists have many oils at their fingertips, but they never mix or use them until they have worked out a prescription for the receiver's individual needs.

Mixing oils is a skilled art, but there are simple recipes, such as those suggested throughout this book, that you can use at home to deal with specific problems from muscular aches and pains to headaches and stress. With potent essential oils it is far better to use less, rather than more, so if in doubt start the massage with a carrier oil such as sweet almond to which you have added 2–3 drops of just one essential oil. Lavender, rosemary and geranium are good, all-purpose oils, or you could use chamomile for particularly sensitive skin.

There is a wide variety of oils available – make sure you choose the right one for your partner.

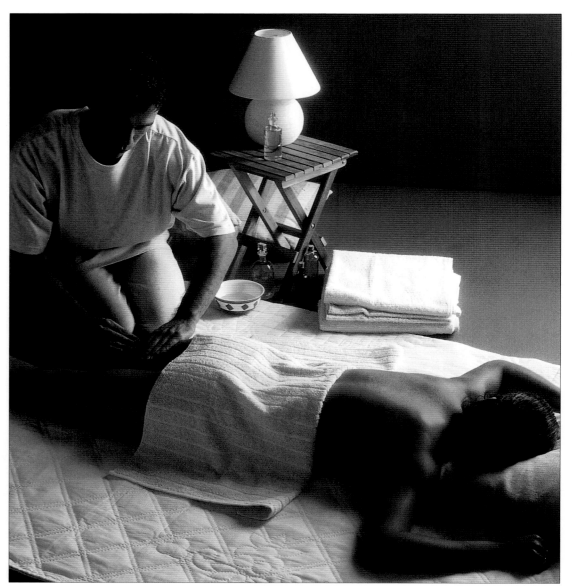

Create a warm, relaxing environment with soft lighting and a comfortable base for your partner to lie on. Play gentle music in the background, and warm the towels before you begin.

GIVING THE MASSAGE

- Before you give a massage to a partner, try out the movements on parts of your own body to get a sense of how the strokes should feel and how much pressure to use.
- Always warm your hands before you begin to apply the oil.
- If the part of the body you're working on is particularly hairy or the skin is very dry, you will need to apply more oil.
- Massage movements should be slow and gentle to help relaxation and eliminate tension which tightens the muscles.
- Remember that the movements should flow into each other. If you find that you have missed out a step or gone on to the wrong part of the body, don't panic. Finish the part you are working on before going back to it, or leave it out altogether rather than interrupting the flow of the massage.
- When you give the massage, make sure you are relaxed and comfortable, as well as your partner, or you will transmit your own tensions and it will not be an effective massage.
- Try to maintain contact with your partner's body as much as possible; even as you move into a different position, try to keep a hand on their body.
- Keep your touch light and sensitive. Remember that your hands are the main channel of communication during the massage.

Keep the oil in an easy dispenser or bowl so you don't have to worry about lids during the massage. But keep the oil covered in some way, as essential oils will quickly evaporate.

RECEIVING THE MASSAGE

Bear the following points in mind when you are planning to have an aromatherapy massage so that you get the most benefit from the treatment.

Before the massage
- Have a cool shower or wash: don't soak in a hot bath, or the oils will immediately seep into the skin.
- Don't use an underarm deodorant or body spray before the treatment, as this will block the effect of the oils.
- Don't have a large meal just before an aromatherapy massage as the body's systems will have to work too hard at digesting to be thoroughly relaxed.
- Don't drink alcohol before a treatment.

- Don't have a massage if you have 'flu or a fever or any serious condition. Wait until you are over the worst, then let an aromatherapy treatment help restore your system's balance.

After the massage
- Lie still for at least 5 minutes before getting up at the end of the treatment.
- Drink a glass of still water immediately after a treatment.
- Don't bathe or shower for at least 12 hours after a treatment to allow the oils to be absorbed by the skin and begin the all-important work of detoxifying the body.
- Drink plenty of water for the rest of the day as the kidneys will be active in eliminating toxins.
- Avoid alcohol for at least 12 hours after the treatment to give the body a chance to detoxify.

Begin the massage with long, calm, flowing strokes to relax your partner both physically and psychologically.

PREPARATION AND EQUIPMENT FOR MASSAGE

A successful massage benefits and relaxes both body and mind, and careful preparation prior to the session helps to achieve this aim. This involves creating a natural and nurturing ambience, as well as having everything you need to hand. Your preparation will give you confidence and trust in your abilities, and your partner will instinctively feel safe in your hands, knowing that you value and respect their comfort and needs. In an atmosphere of mutual relaxation, your massage can proceed in a calm and serene manner.

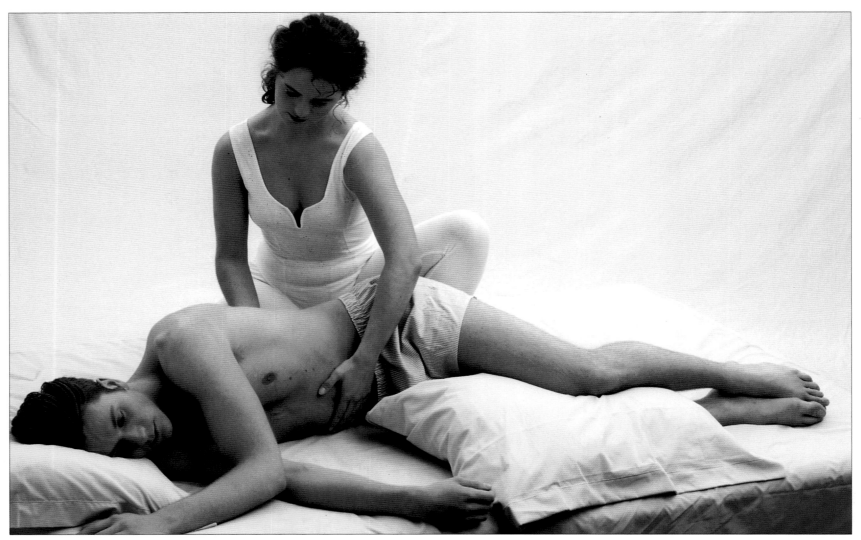

A futon is ideal for massage, but a foam rubber mattress placed on the floor is a suitable alternative. Wear clean, light, comfortable clothing that is not too tight when giving a massage. Remember that giving a massage is quite energetic and you will get warmer as you proceed.

Have all materials and equipment ready in advance of the massage, including tissues and oils.

THE SETTING

Most rooms can be easily converted into a peaceful setting. Soft, diffused lighting will enhance a tranquil mood. Ensure that the room you choose is warm and draught-free, as body temperature is likely to drop rapidly while lying still, especially when your partner is covered in oil. As the giver of the massage, be aware of the discrepancy between your body temperature and that of your partner. Wear light, comfortable clothing while giving the massage.

Privacy and quiet is essential to relaxation during massage. Pick a time when you will not be disturbed or hurried, bearing in mind that a complete massage may last between an hour and an hour-and-a-half.

All sheets, towels and pillowcases should be freshly laundered for each session.

EQUIPMENT

Have a pile of fresh, clean towels and sheets ready for use. Cover the surface your partner will be lying on with a sheet. Have several pillows or thinly folded towels ready to place beneath the body to ease areas of tension. If the massage will take place at floor level, use cushions to kneel or sit on for your own comfort.

The massage base must be firm, comfortable and supportive. A futon or foam rubber mattress is ideal, or you can provide adequate padding with folded blankets. Beds are generally too soft unless you are stroking only very lightly. Ensure that the area surrounding the massage base is uncluttered so you have maximum freedom of movement.

Have all your aromatherapy materials and equipment ready for use before the session begins. Under some circumstances it may be preferable to use the selected essential oils in a vaporizer rather than blend them with the massage oil. Tissues or small towels should be available for wiping oil from your hands, or for your partner's convenience. If you are concerned about oil stains, place a thin rubber sheet under the massage sheet, or a beautician's tissue couch roll or a bath towel over the top of the sheet. If essential oil is accidentally spilt on clothing, dab it off quickly with a tissue. It will soon evaporate but it may leave a stain, so rinse out clothing in warm soapy water.

PERSONAL HYGIENE

This is very important for both participants. Make certain you come to the session freshly showered, with clean nails, hands and feet. Wipe your hands after massaging the feet before proceeding with strokes on other parts of the body. Always wash your hands thoroughly at the end of each massage session.

Wooden massage tools in various shapes are particularly useful for self-massage.

THE BASIC TECHNIQUES OF MASSAGE

The following pages introduce the basic techniques of massage, which will help you build up a flowing sequence of strokes and enable you to bring a harmonious state of relaxation and invigoration to your partner.

KEEPING YOUR PARTNER COMFORTABLE

Use warmed, fresh, clean towels to cover your partner during massage. The towels will prevent the loss of body heat once the oil has been applied and the person is lying still. They also ensure your partner's modesty is respected. Move the towels as needed while applying your strokes, leaving uncovered only the area on which you are working during the massage.

1 Ideally you should use one large bath towel to cover the whole body, and two medium-sized towels to add further warmth to the upper body and the feet. Tuck the towel snugly around both feet.

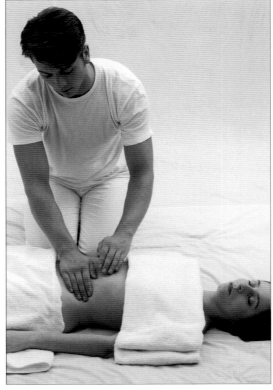

2 When massaging the abdomen, peel back the large towel and cover the breasts with a folded towel. Do not leave the chest and breasts exposed.

3 Once you are working on the legs, ensure that the upper body stays warm by covering it with an extra towel. Fold the large towel over so that only the leg on which you are working remains exposed.

4 When your partner turns over, hold the towel up between you both, and then let it drop softly down on the other side of the body.

BEGINNING THE MASSAGE

After you have decided on the blend of essential oils you will be using for the massage, give your partner time to undress and make themselves comfortable and relaxed while you mix the oils. Take a few moments to calm yourself and centre your thoughts before you begin. Your first contact with your partner should be steady and reassuring.

1 Rub a little of your chosen blend of oil into the palms of your hands and spread it over the area you intend to massage with the flat of the hands, in smooth, flowing motions. For the initial stroke, the flowing motion should define the contours of the whole of the area you intend to massage. While integrating the whole surface of the body, this stroke also warms the muscles and prepares them for subsequent massage techniques. The integration stroke is usually a large, flowing and continuous motion, which is repeated 3–5 times for full effect.

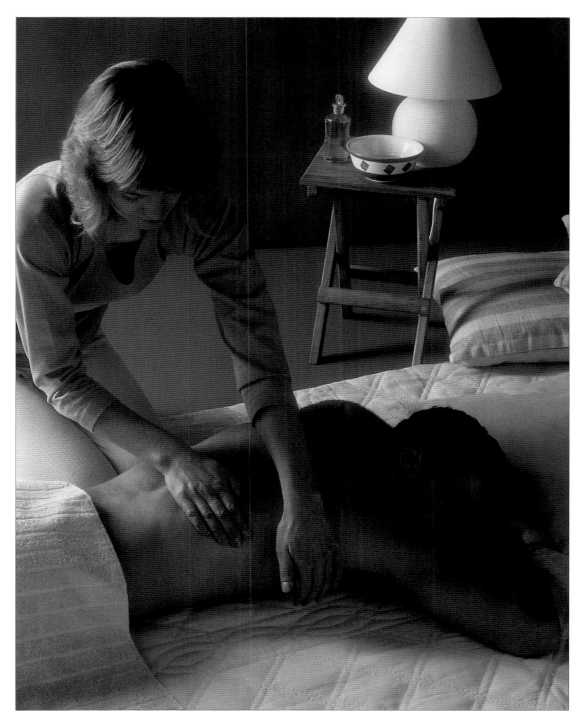

Arrange the mattress or futon on which your partner is to lie so that there is sufficient space for you to move freely around it.

EFFLEURAGE

Effleurage is the first and main stroke of massage. It prepares the body's soft tissues and warms the muscles for all deeper movements. It is also used to follow up more vigorous strokes such as kneading and friction, in order to soothe and relax an area that has just been massaged. Effleurage simply means "stroking", and is a free-flowing, continuous movement made with the flat of one or, more usually, both hands at a steady pressure.

Effleurage strokes have a calming and almost hypnotic effect on the body, allowing a sense of trust to develop so that the recipient can relax both physically and psychologically. The strokes can be applied with a light to medium pressure, with the whole hand in contact with the skin. When applied in a movement up towards the heart, these strokes benefit the cardiovascular system (the heart and network of blood vessels) and the lymphatic system by boosting the circulation of blood and lymph around the body. A lighter movement has a calming effect on the function of the nervous system.

While making the strokes, the hands should be completely relaxed so that they mould themselves into the body's contours and define its shape. Effleurage has a fluid quality so that the strokes flow around the body and never finish abruptly.

FANNING

Fanning is an effleurage movement that can be applied to many areas of the body, including the back, chest, legs and arms. It is an excellent stroke to follow on from larger preparatory movements and can be used to stretch and manipulate tension away from the muscles. Fanning can be applied either as a series of shorter movements for remedial effect or in larger, more flowing motions for sensual and soothing effects. Use a steady pressure for the upward stroke and keep the movement slow and relaxed.

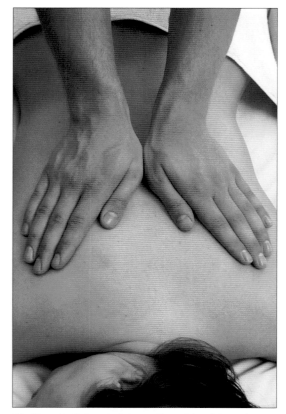

1 Place both hands flat on either side of the spine with the fingers together, pointing straight up towards the head. Keeping the whole hand in contact with the skin, stroke with an even pressure for about 15 cm/6 in up the back. Now let your hands flow outwards in a fanning motion, moving away from each other towards the sides of the ribcage.

2 Shape your hands to the sides of the body, then draw the hands down before sliding them lightly around and towards their original position alongside the spine. Now stroke further up the back.

CONTINUOUS CIRCLE STROKES

Continuous circle strokes add a sensual, relaxing and soporific element to the massage. If applied at a more vigorous pace and with slightly firmer pressure, they are excellent for warming the superficial layers of tissue and for releasing tension. These effleurage strokes can be used on any broad expanse of the body, such as the sides of the ribcage, the back and the thighs, when they are applied in a flowing, unbroken motion. Continuous circle strokes also form the main preparatory strokes on the abdomen.

2 While your left hand continues to make a full circle, the right hand lifts up and passes over the top of the moving left hand.

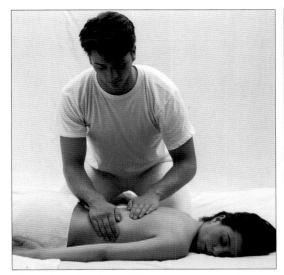

1 Lay both hands parallel to each other and flat on the area you intend to massage. The hands should be both flexible and soft enough to mould into the body's contours. Begin to slide both hands in the same direction in a circular motion.

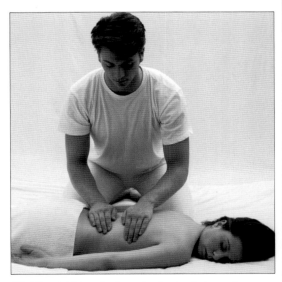

3 The right hand returns to the body to perform a half-circle stroke before lifting off again to let the left hand complete the next full circular motion.

KNEADING

Kneading is one of the most satisfying strokes in massage both to give and to receive, because it takes hold of the muscle and moves it about, creating greater flexibility and suppleness. To knead well, the hands should be dextrous and pliable; the motion is similar to the action of a baker kneading dough.

Kneading is a lifting, squeezing and rolling movement that passes the flesh from one hand to the other. It has a rhythmic, circular motion and should be applied with the wrists and shoulders relaxed, and the arms held at a distance from the body. Stand or kneel on the opposite side of the body, so that your fingers are pointing downwards as you work.

Kneading is a good stroke to apply on muscular and fleshy areas such as the calves, thighs, buttocks and waist after they have been relaxed and warmed by effleurage. It benefits the muscles by releasing underlying tension, breaking down fat deposits and toxins trapped in the tissues and aiding the exchange of tissue fluids. Always follow up kneading with effleurage strokes to soothe the area and boost the blood and lymph circulation so that released toxins can be properly eliminated from the body.

FRICTION AND PRESSURE STROKES

Friction and pressure strokes work on releasing tension by pushing the muscle down towards the bone and then stretching it. Apply after kneading on fleshy areas, or following effleurage wherever the bone is close to the surface of the skin, such as on the hands, feet, face or alongside the spine. A pressure stroke is made by leaning your weight steadily into muscle or connective tissue. The heel of the hand, thumb pads, finger pads, knuckles and forearm can all be used. The pressure must always be applied and released slowly and sensitively.

2 By keeping the whole hand relaxed but applying direct pressure into the heel, these circular motions will ease tension from the muscles of the buttocks.

3 The small surfaces of the thumb pads are able to penetrate into those areas where muscles and tendons are attached to bone, for example alongside the spine. Painful tight spots can be eased by leaning weight into the thumbs while the hands remain relaxed on the body, and then making a good firm sliding motion up each side of the spine.

1 The heel of the hand provides a broad, flat surface with which to add pressure during massage, and it is particularly effective in stretching and draining muscle in tight areas such as the lower back and thighs. Shift the weight in the hands into the heels and use in alternating, circular motions – one hand following the other in a continuous flow of movement. The pressure should be applied in the upward and outward half of the slide, but decreased in the last half of the circle as the hands glide softly around to repeat the stroke.

4 Support the back of your partner's hand with your fingers and use small and continuously alternating thumb circles over the palms and wrists to remove stiffness. To achieve the correct movement in these strokes, you must rotate the thumbs from their base joint.

5 Finger pad pressure can be applied to release tension from under bone, such as the ridge of the skull. The pressure must be applied slowly to allow your partner time to relax. Slowly rotate your fingertips on one area at a time. Then release the pressure gradually before moving to the next spot.

PERCUSSION

Percussion strokes include a variety of invigorating movements that briskly strike fleshy and muscular areas of the body to produce a toning and stimulating effect on the skin. They are performed with one hand following the other in a series of rapid and rhythmic movements, helping to draw the blood towards the skin's surface and leaving it with a warm and healthy glow. The rapid action also dispels tension and rids the tissues of excess fluid and fatty deposits. To achieve the best results, keep your shoulders, wrists and hands relaxed, and bounce your hands immediately back off the skin the moment they make contact.

The invigorating effects of percussion help to enliven the body after the euphoric effects of other massage strokes, but they may not be suitable to use if your partner is in a particularly sensitive or vulnerable mood. Percussion strokes should never be applied over varicose veins or directly on top of bone.

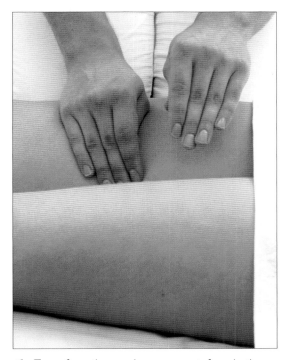

1 To perform the cupping movement, form both hands into a softly cupped shape by keeping your fingers straight but bent at the lower knuckles; at the same time draw the thumbs close into the palms. This should create an airtight vacuum in the centre of your palms, which exerts suction on the skin during the rapid cupping action. Using the palms to make contact, briskly strike and flick off the skin, one hand following the other in quick succession over fleshy areas.

2 Hacking uses the same fast rhythmic motion as cupping, but contact with the skin is made from the sides of the hands, one following the other in quick succession. The wrists and fingers should be relaxed and the palms of each hand should face each other with only about 2.5 cm/1 in between them. Hacking tones and stimulates all fleshy areas, and works particularly well on the buttocks, thighs and tops of the shoulders.

3 For the pummelling stroke, keep your shoulders and wrists relaxed and make loose fists in order to pummel over the fleshy parts of your partner's body. Contact with the skin is made with the sides of the hands. Apply the stroke in the same brisk fashion as the previous percussion strokes, letting one hand after the other pummel over the area you are massaging. This stroke, applied to the thighs and buttocks, is excellent for helping to break down cellulite.

APPLYING THE CORRECT SEQUENCE OF STROKES

The following sequence of strokes on the calf muscles of the leg shows the order in which the basic techniques of massage should be applied to create a relaxing and invigorating effect. This sequence can be used, as appropriate, on any part of the body.

1 *Effleurage*: Soothing strokes made with the flat of the hands will warm and loosen tense calf muscles and prepare them for deeper strokes.

2 *Kneading*: Knead the calf muscles to invigorate the muscles and help them to contract. Follow up with some soft strokes.

3 *Friction*: Press your thumb pads sensitively into the muscle tissue using alternating thumb circle friction strokes. This will stretch and release a deeper level of tension. Work thoroughly over the whole area.

4 *Vibrating*: Gently sink your fingertips into the calf muscle and vibrate it rapidly. Let your hands mould into the shape of the lower leg as you follow the vibrating action with flowing effleurage.

5 *Cupping*: Cup the calf briskly to stimulate the blood circulation and tone the skin and the muscles. Apply the cupping motion up and down the lower leg several times.

6 *Hacking*: Use the hacking stroke over the bulk of the calf muscles for further toning, and to aid the elimination of excess tissue fluids. Do not strike the back of the knee. *Stroking*: Gently stroke over the calf as in step 1, to harmonize the previous massage movements and to boost both the blood and lymph circulation towards the heart.

OILS IN THERAPY

Aromatherapy treats both mind and body, working mainly on the nervous system, and is able both to relax and stimulate. When it is used in massage, the highly potent essential oils penetrate the body via the skin and are also inhaled as the treatment progresses. While the techniques and strokes of massage can ease pain or tension from stiff and aching muscles, boost a sluggish circulation or eliminate toxins, at the same time the nurturing touch of the hands on the body soothes away mental stress and restores emotional equilibrium.

The use of essential oils in therapy can help to alleviate specific symptoms, but can also help to promote a more balanced and healthy lifestyle. There is less likelihood of succumbing to everyday illnesses such as colds, and of suffering from the effects of stress. A balanced state of mind promotes vitality and a better ability to cope with potentially difficult events or situations, such as a crisis at work, an interview, or even a visit to the dentist. The use of aromatherapy can also stimulate the immune system, avoiding the run down feeling which can lead to flu-like symptoms or general weariness. The following pages are a guide to the use of oils in the alleviation of complaints such as headache, nausea and the symptoms of flu, stress and bad circulation.

Massage with essential oils works both physically and psychologically to relax and stimulate the nervous system.

EASING HEADACHES AND MIGRAINES

Most headaches are caused by tension, but occasionally they are the result of an allergic reaction to food or a symptom of an ailment such as sinusitis. Whatever the cause, gentle massage at the earliest moment can help to stop headaches from getting a tight grip. Compresses are another option: a cold compress of lavender or geranium across the forehead will provide pleasant relief, or for tension in the neck sandalwood can be helpful.

RELEASING CONSTRICTED MUSCLES

It is thought that tension headaches are caused by a change in blood pressure brought about when muscles tense and restrict blood flow. The main areas of muscular tension are the shoulders, neck and below the ridge of the skull.

RECOMMENDED ESSENTIAL OILS

To relieve a tension headache or migraine:
Lavender.

If the headache is the result of overwork, anger or worry:
Chamomile or marjoram.
For a sharp, piercing pain;
if the head feels hot:
Peppermint.

For a feeling of lethargy and despondency:
Lemon or rosemary.

To relieve the symptoms of colds and sinusitis:
Eucalyptus.

At the earliest stages of a migraine, blend 2 drops rosemary, 1 drop each marjoram and clary sage.

1 Rest one hand on each shoulder for a few moments, then, anchoring your fingers over the top of the shoulders, roll and squeeze the muscles in a kneading action, using the heels of your hands. Work out to the edge of the shoulders and down the tops of the arms.

2 Place one hand across the forehead and the other across the nape of the neck. Ask your partner to drop her head into your hand and breathe gently, imagining that she is releasing tension with each out-going breath. Gently squeeze the neck muscles between the fingers and heel of your hand.

3 Still supporting the forehead, use the thumb pad of the other hand to press upwards into the hollow at the top of the spine. Apply gentle pressure for a steady count of five, then release.

4 Loosen the constricted muscles under the base of the skull by massaging beneath the bony ridge, working from the top of the spine to the outer edge of the skull. Change hands to massage the other side. Ease scalp tension by rotating the fingertips of both hands in small circles all over the head.

STRETCHING THE NECK MUSCLES

Tense neck muscles can be eased through gentle stretching. It is important to make sure your partner is lying perfectly straight before you begin.

1 Slip both hands under your partner's shoulders, with your fingers resting at the top of the spine and your palms supporting the back of the neck. Ask your partner to relax her neck into your hands, then pull them steadily upwards to stretch and lengthen the neck away from the shoulders. Raise her head slightly as your hands pass under the hairline and up the back of the head.

2 Cup the head in your hands, with your fingers resting on the neck and your thumbs lying gently against the sides of the face. Encouraging your partner to relax completely, lift the head slightly, then roll it gently to the right and to the left. Repeat this action several times.

DRAWING OUT THE PAIN

These four techniques all involve applying pressure then releasing it, to relax muscles and lift the pain of a tension headache away from the head.

1 Settle your hands lightly around your partner's scalp for a few moments. Keeping your hands in the cupped position, lift them slowly away from the head as if they were drawing out the pain.

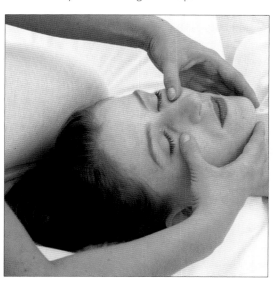

3 Working from inner to outer edge, apply a press/release motion under the ridge of both eyebrows using the tips of your index fingers. Then use your thumb pads to press/release over the top of the cheekbones, working out from the nose to the edge of the temples.

2 Cup your hands around the head again, placing your thumbs between the eyebrows. Apply gentle pressure with your thumbs for a count of five, then release the pressure.

4 Briskly rub your hands together to create heat, then softly lay your slightly cupped palms over the eyes for a count of five to soothe and relax the eye muscles. Withdraw your hands slowly.

CALMING ANXIETY AND STRESS

Aromatherapy and massage provide excellent antidotes to the symptoms of anxiety and stress. A prolonged state of anxiety can deplete vital energy from the body, leading to a general state of nervousness and tension. While essential oils will soothe and comfort, massage strokes will return a sense of physical reality, helping to calm the anxiety.

Anxiety can be alleviated with a combination of uplifting and calming oils, used in an aromatic bath or blended into a massage oil. Whichever oils you choose, use two relaxing oils to one uplifting one.

To prevent undue stress, when you find yourself in a potentially stressful situation try simply inhaling one of your favourite oils at regular intervals. Alternatively, you could put a couple of drops of a relaxing oil such as lavender or geranium in a vaporizer in your room or office to help keep you feeling more relaxed and calm.

RECOMMENDED ESSENTIAL OILS

To aid relaxation and reduce the effects of stress:
Lavender, geranium, marjoram.

To comfort and lift the spirits:
Basil, clary sage, ylang ylang.

If the anxiety attack causes a digestive upset:
Neroli.

To alleviate a sense of alienation:
Sandalwood, rosewood or frankincense.

Blend 5 drops each basil, neroli and lavender with 15 ml/1 tbsp carrier oil to use as a restorative bath oil.

SOOTHING AWAY STRESS

Releasing tension from the brow, temples, jaw and neck will help to calm the mind.

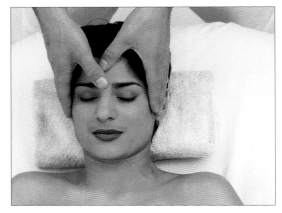

1 Using your thumbs in the centre of the forehead, stroke one after the other in short, firm slides, to ease the tension from the area between, and directly above, the eyebrows.

3 Placing your fingers around the back of the head, use the thumbs to stroke in soft, circular motions over the temples.

2 Using the palms and fingers, brush your hands soothingly in alternating motions from one side of the forehead to the other. With the fingers of your right hand pointing to the left temple, draw your hand lightly across the brow, before lifting it off to let your left hand repeat the motion from the right temple.

4 Releasing and extending the neck will loosen constricted muscles. Place both hands, fingers pointing downwards, along each side of the top of the spine. Ask your partner to breathe deeply and relax her neck and head back into your hands. Pull your hands gently, with the fingertips slightly indented into the tissue, up the back of the neck and out from under the head.

THE SOLAR PLEXUS STROKE

This is a marvellous way of unlocking tension by calming the main nerves that run through this area in the centre of the body. Use your left hand (for calming) to stroke the solar plexus (located just below the breast bone) in anti-clockwise circles. Close your eyes as you do this and try to empty your mind of the anxious thoughts that are making you feel tense, concentrating instead on what you are doing. This calming action can help soothe you even if you do it through your clothes, but the effect is enhanced if you use a relaxing essential oil on the skin, such as lavender or geranium. Try it while your bath is running, or when lying in bed before you go to sleep.

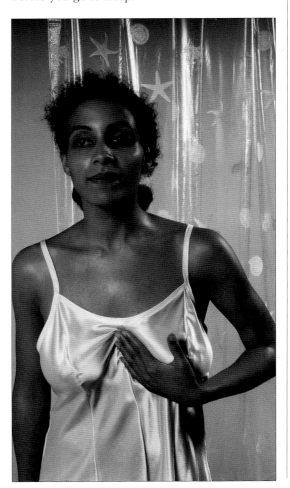

PULSING THE JOINTS

Passive movements to loosen and relax the joints of the body will help to release tension. It is important to encourage your partner to give up the control of movement and weight of her limbs into your hands, thereby enabling her to trust you and free her tension. Gently rotate, wiggle, stretch and rock the joints of the body in line with their natural movement. Encourage your partner to breathe into these areas to allow a greater sense of connection to her body. You can follow up these passive movements with massage on the arms, hands, legs and feet to release tension. Never try to force someone into relaxing, however, and always respect their level of tension.

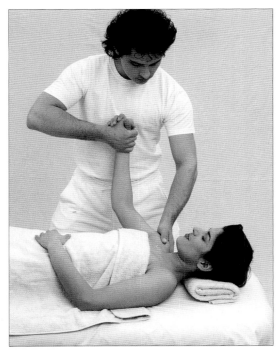

1 Keeping the elbow slightly flexed, lift the arm away from the body. To secure your hold, clasp the wrist and hand and slip your thumb between your partner's thumb and index finger. Place your other hand supportively behind the shoulder. Rock the arm gently so that the movement travels up into the shoulder joint. Lift and lower the arm as you rock it to encourage a complete release of tension.

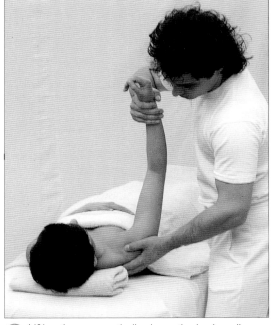

2 Lifting the arm vertically above the body, pull gently upwards to create an easy stretch in the joint before slowly releasing the traction. Then, with the elbow slightly flexed, bounce the arm gently up and down into the shoulder socket, and against the support of your hand.

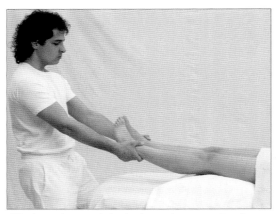

3 A gentle stretch in the legs releases tension from the hips and pelvis. Positioning yourself below your partner's feet, clasp the back of both ankles with your hands. Lean back in your own body to pull her legs towards you, and then slowly and easily release this traction.

INSOMNIA

Sleeplessness is a common response to stress, as your mind and body refuse to let go enough to give you the rest that you need. The resulting disturbed and restless night leaves you more prone to stress and anxiety, and a vicious cycle can be created. Learning to relax has to be built into a daily pattern based on a healthy diet, regular exercise and a calming routine to wind down before bedtime.

I t is important to reduce your intake of stimulating drinks such as tea or coffee, and to avoid eating late at night. It is also helpful to create a relaxing ritual to prepare for falling asleep, with a pleasantly warm evening bath to which you have added your chosen blend of sedative oils. Just experiencing a fragrance that you enjoy will help you to unwind after a long day.

RECOMMENDED ESSENTIAL OILS

Chamomile, clary sage, lavender, marjoram, mandarin, neroli, orange, rose, rosewood and sandalwood.

For sleeplessness following bad dreams: Blend frankincense, lemon or ylang ylang with any of the above oils.

Blends for relaxing bath oils: 4 drops rose and 3 drops sandalwood or 5 drops lavender and 3 drops ylang ylang.

A GENTLE WAVE

The following sequence of strokes washes over the limbs and extremities of the body in outward flowing motions, creating a gentle stream of movement. The soft, downward pulling strokes have a hypnotic and sedative effect, which will calm the emotions and quiet an overactive mind, thereby helping to induce relaxation and sleep.

As you apply the strokes, draw your hands down on the inhalation and pause briefly on the exhalation. This almost imperceptible pause in the motion will create a lovely wave-like feeling, rather than a straight, pulling effect. Each sequence should be performed up to five times on each part of the body.

1 Place one hand over the top of the chest, and the other over the muscles on the back of the shoulder, so that the fingers point towards the centre of the body. As you breathe in, pull your hands steadily outwards to the edge of the shoulder and down to just below the joint. Pause briefly as you exhale, letting your hands rest and lightly cradle the top of the arm.

2 Adjust your position so that you can continue the pulling motion down the length of the arm. As you breathe in, pull both hands down to just below the elbow joint. Relax as you breathe out, then continue the slide down the forearm and below the wrist with your next inhalation.

3 Draw your hands over both sides of your partner's hand and fingers, taking your stroke out beyond the body as the hand settles back on to the mattress. Repeat steps 1 to 3 on the other side of the body.

4 Lay both hands slightly above the pelvic girdle to cradle the side of the body. Pull both hands down over the hip socket as you inhale, separating them as they reach the thigh in order to hold each side of the leg; rest briefly as you exhale. With the next inhalation, draw your hands down the leg to just below the knee.

5 Continue this wave-like motion down the lower leg to just below the ankle, then – sliding one hand under the foot with the other on top of the foot – pull gently and steadily out over the toes. Repeat this sequence of strokes on the other side of the body.

SEDATING STROKES ON THE LEGS AND FEET

Finish the sequence with this soothing movement until you feel your partner is relaxed.

1 Using the flat of both hands, softly stroke down the legs from the thighs until your hands pass over and out of the feet. Repeat the movement as many times as you like to allow your partner to relax.

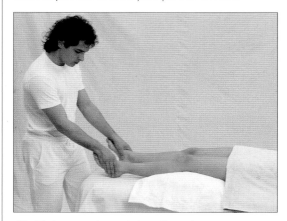

2 To increase the sedative effect of your strokes, complete these sequences with a still, calm hold of your hands over the front of both feet. This will draw the energy down the body, bringing a sense of balance and equilibrium.

ALLEVIATING THE SYMPTOMS OF A COLD

While a cold will normally run its course, combining self-massage with aromatherapy treatment can bring considerable relief from the symptoms. Adding the recommended essential oils to a vaporizer or bowl of steaming water will enable you to inhale their remedial effects, helping to clear the head and soothe the throat and chest, while boosting the immune system.

The foremost treatment for a cold is plenty of rest, which allows the immune system to fight off the viral infection. In the normal course of events a cold usually takes about a week to clear, but if the symptoms persist longer than this, or worsen, it may be advisable to consult your doctor. In the meantime, drink plenty of fluids and increase your intake of fruit and vegetables to help cleanse the body of mucus.

A large number of essential oils can be comforting and helpful in relieving cold symptoms. Tea tree is perhaps the most useful, while eucalyptus is invaluable for relieving a blocked nose and head. All oils are to some extent antiseptic and will assist in preventing the spread of infection. Because most colds present a mixture of symptoms, you should choose one oil for each symptom, then add tea tree to the blend.

INHALING ESSENTIAL OILS

Pour your blended oils into a bowl of hot water and, as they vaporize, inhale the steam as deeply as possible. The oils will begin to decongest blocked nasal passages and soothe the cold symptoms. If you hold a towel over your head this will delay the effects of evaporation. Be careful to place the bowl in a safe position.

RECOMMENDED ESSENTIAL OILS

For the early stages of a cold:
Nutmeg.

For a runny cold:
Ginger.

For bronchitis:
Cedarwood, eucalyptus, frankincense, neroli, orange, peppermint, rosemary, sandalwood.

To loosen catarrh:
Cypress, frankincense, jasmine, lemon, black pepper, sandalwood.

To free congestion:
Frankincense, lemon, eucalyptus.

To boost the immune system:
Bergamot, grapefruit, lavender, lemon, marjoram, rosewood.

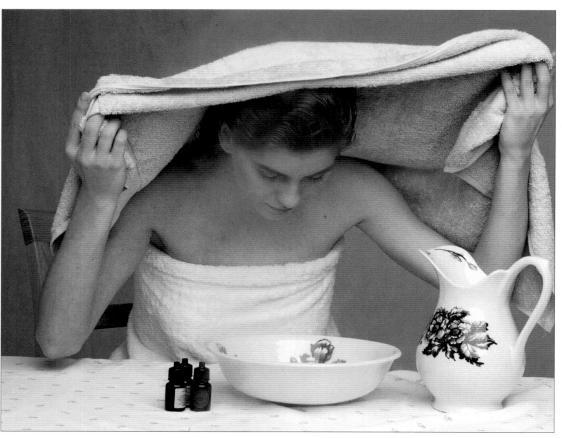

Try a steam inhalation with essential oils to treat nasal congestion or to relieve the pain of sinusitis.

SELF-MASSAGE FOR A COLD

After a steam inhalation, apply some self-massage strokes and pressure on specific points to relieve blocked sinuses.

1 Massage all over your brow, starting from the centre and working out with small circular motions from your fingertips.

2 Release pressure from the sinus passages by pinching along the ridge of your eyebrows with your thumbs and index fingers, starting on the inside corners and working, step by step, to the outer edges.

3 Stroke your temples with your fingertips, moving them over the area in circular motions. This will alleviate the stuffiness that can lead to headaches.

4 To relieve congested nasal passages, use your fingertips to press gently into each side of the outer rim of the nostrils at the edge of the cheekbones. Hold for a count of five and then slowly release the pressure.

5 The small indentations beneath the ridges of the cheekbones indicate the location of some of the sinus passages. Apply thumb pressure slowly up into the hollows. Hold for a count of five and release. This will help clear the head.

MASSAGE THERAPIES TO AID DIGESTION

Emotional tension can cause us to tighten our abdominal muscles and reduce our breathing in order to avoid the experience of painful or uncomfortable feelings. If we are unable to assimilate those emotions, or express them appropriately, they can manifest themselves as physical disorders, particularly playing havoc with the digestive system.

RECOMMENDED ESSENTIAL OILS

To accelerate a sluggish digestion:
Peppermint, black pepper, palmarosa, nutmeg.

For flatulence:
Bergamot, black pepper, fennel, ginger, lemon, marjoram, neroli, nutmeg, peppermint, rosemary.

To soothe colicky pain:
Bergamot, chamomile, clary sage, ginger, cypress, lemon, orange, peppermint, sandalwood.

Constipation:
Black pepper, fennel, ginger, marjoram, neroli, nutmeg, orange, peppermint, rose.

Diarrhoea:
Cypress, chamomile, ginger, lemon, orange, peppermint, black pepper.

A blend for indigestion, colic and flatulence:
1 drop peppermint, 3 drops each of ginger, lemon and bergamot.

Blends for a relaxing compress:
To a bowl of hot water, add 2 drops orange and 3 drops peppermint, or 3 drops chamomile and 2 drops orange.

The key to eliminating indigestion caused by tension is to allow our bodies to let go of such worries and anxieties, and aromatherapy can help a great deal to achieve this. One of the easiest ways to use oils in this context is to disperse them in a bowl of hot water, then make a hot compress and place it over the abdomen, keeping the area warm for up to 10 minutes.

HOLDING AND BREATHING

Still, calm holds over the abdominal area will encourage deeper breathing, allowing the release of pent-up emotions and stress. The following holds will all help to promote relaxation and eliminate tension, enabling the digestive tract to function properly.

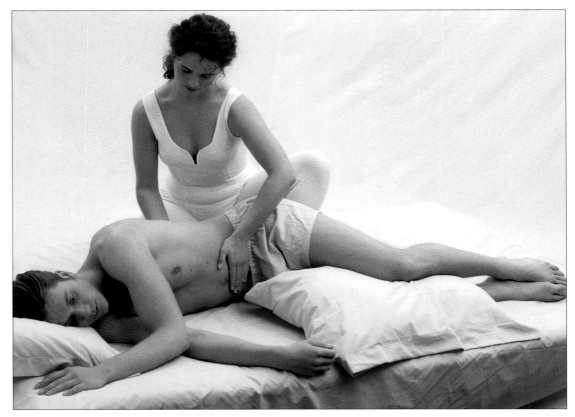

1 If your partner is under extreme stress and is experiencing abdominal pain, ask him to lie on his side with his knees drawn up slightly. Put pillows under his head and between his knees to create a feeling of security. Place one hand over the lower back and the other on his belly, and ask him to breathe slowly and deeply from the abdomen. When the abdominal muscles are relaxed, rub the belly with gentle clockwise strokes.

2 Ask your partner to lie on his back with his knees raised. Place one hand under the small of his back and ask him to drop the weight of his pelvis towards your hand. Place your other hand over the abdomen so that its warmth helps to dissolve constriction in the muscles. Then ask your partner to direct his breathing towards your hands and to imagine that each breath is helping the belly to expand and release tension.
Then move your top hand to hold different parts of the abdomen.

3 Encourage deep but gentle breathing in the abdomen and solar plexus region by placing one hand behind the back and the other over the top of the abdomen to encourage the release of tension that can lead to digestive problems. As the area relaxes, gently massage the abdomen with circular strokes of your palm.

RELIEVING ABDOMINAL CRAMP

Passive movements can also be used to reduce the tension which leads to abdominal tightness and pain. You can help to relieve cramp in your partner's belly by pushing his knees towards him. Ask your partner to bend his knees, keeping his feet on the mattress. Adjust your own posture so that you can lean your weight forward as you perform this passive movement. Encourage your partner to give up to you all control of the weight and movement of his legs and concentrate on breathing more deeply. Slowly push the knees towards the trunk of the body, taking care not to force them beyond their natural point of resistance. Help to lower your partner's feet to the mattress, then repeat the movement twice more.

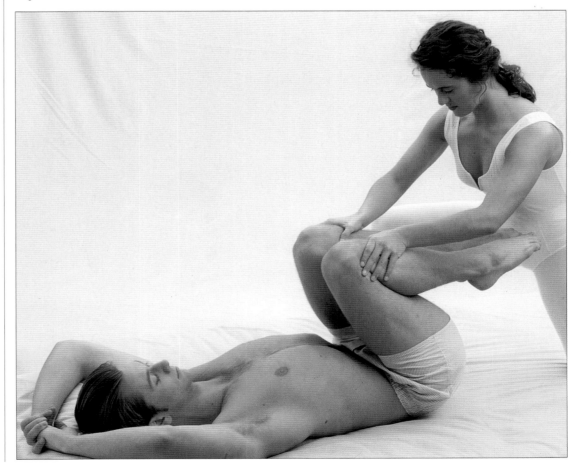

IMPROVING CIRCULATION

A healthy circulatory system is vital to the well-being of both mind and body. Massage with stimulating essential oils, combined with a healthy diet and exercise, is an excellent way of boosting both blood and lymph circulation in order to promote health and vitality.

The circulatory system is divided into two parts: blood circulation, pumped by the heart, and lymph fluid circulation, moved by muscle action. The lymphatic system carries waste products to the lymph nodes, which act as filters to prevent harmful substances from entering the bloodstream, and is an important part of the body's immune defence system.

Poor circulation may be caused by hereditary factors, but it is also affected by a sedentary lifestyle, smoking, an unhealthy diet or emotional stress and tension. A sluggish circulation will cause a depletion of vital nutrients in the body, leading to exhaustion, ill-health, and even depression as toxins build up and the elimination process is impeded. Stimulating essential oils can help to counteract this process and tone up the circulatory system.

RECOMMENDED ESSENTIAL OILS

To stimulate circulation:
Benzoin, black pepper, cedarwood, cypress, eucalyptus, geranium, grapefruit, lemon, mandarin, neroli, rose, rosemary.

To detoxify:
Black pepper, eucalyptus, fennel.

Blend one or more of the stimulant oils with one of the detoxifying oils listed above to treat the problem of poor circulation fully.

BOOSTING AND DRAINING

The signs of a sluggish circulation include pale, mottled or blue-tinged skin, which is usually cold to the touch. The most common areas of poor circulation are the extremities. Lift the limb and apply flowing strokes to boost and drain the blood supply on its return to the heart.

1 Raise your partner's forearm and clasp his hand. Wrap the other hand over the back of the wrist and drain firmly down the arm towards the elbow with a long steady stroke. Glide lightly around the elbow and back up to the wrist. Swap hands to repeat the movement on the inner forearm.

2 Help to increase vitality in the legs and feet by first applying the basic effleurage stroke from the ankle to the back of the knee, with the lower leg in a raised position. Wrap both hands over the back of the ankle, little fingers leading, and firmly stroke up the calf. This position also helps to drain excess water from around puffy ankles.

3 Deeper drainage strokes can be achieved by using your thumbs to stroke, in alternating short slides, from the ankle to just below the back of the knee. Repeat several times.

WARMING UP

Hands and feet that are cold as a result of poor circulation can be warmed up by briskly rubbing them between both hands. The friction produces heat and stimulates the blood supply.

STROKING TOWARDS LYMPH NODES

Gentle, upward effleurage strokes towards the major superficial lymph nodes – such as those in the back of the knee – can assist the lymphatic circulatory system to eliminate toxins from the body, particularly after kneading, friction and deep tissue massage.

BENEFITING THE SKIN

Pale, flaccid skin benefits from the stimulating effects of all percussion strokes. In particular, the suction effect of cupping draws the blood up towards the skin, bringing vital oxygen and nutrients to its peripheral nerve endings and underlying tissues.

VARICOSE VEINS

The return of de-oxygenated blood to the heart from the lower half of the leg is against the pull of gravity, and some veins have valves in them that open and close to prevent back-flow. When a valve is damaged the veins become dilated causing the condition known as varicose veins. This condition can be exacerbated by pregnancy, obesity, or prolonged standing.

It is not advisable to massage directly above or below a varicose vein, but gentle upward-flowing effleurage over the sides of the leg, or away from the damaged vein, will ensure that the area is not neglected during massage. Essential oil blends that improve the circulation will help, but if varicose veins are a result of pregnancy you should not use any oils that are contra-indicated at this time.

DISPERSING CELLULITE AND DETOXIFICATION

Cellulite, which collects mostly on the hips, buttocks and upper arms, is not specifically related to body weight and affects people of all sizes, especially women. It is caused by the accumulation of toxic deposits in the fatty tissues and is detectable by the bumpy "orange peel" look of the skin in these problem areas.

A build-up of cellulite usually results from a sluggish circulation and poor elimination of toxins from the body. To improve the condition it is necessary to use a combination of approaches. Review your diet and cut down on the intake of toxins such as refined carbohydrates, caffeine and alcohol. Increase the amount of fresh vegetables and water. Fennel tea is a natural diuretic which will aid the elimination of toxins. Regular exercise is also important, as it helps the lymphatic system rid the body of waste products.

Massage with the recommended essential oils should become part of your daily routine for 6–8 weeks to help achieve a smooth and healthy skin. Mechanical massage instruments are helpful for this. You can try a quick self-massage several times a day, such as when dressing or after taking a bath or shower. Squeeze and knead the thighs and buttocks, and follow up with a range of percussion movements to shift fatty deposits under the skin.

RECOMMENDED ESSENTIAL OILS

To stimulate and detoxify:
Black pepper, eucalyptus, fennel.

To stimulate circulation and prevent water retention:
Geranium, lemon, grapefruit.

Blend 3 drops lemon, 2 drops geranium, 2 drops fennel and 1 drop black pepper in 10 ml/2 tsp carrier oil.

SELF-MASSAGE

1 Hand-held massage instruments such as this wooden six-ball roller are ideal for making the circular pressure motions that help to smooth out cellulite spots on the thighs.

2 Hack, cup and pummel the thighs briskly to tone the area and revitalize the blood circulation.

CELLULITE REDUCTION MASSAGE

If cellulite is a problem, focus your attention on the problem areas of the thighs and buttocks when giving a massage to boost the blood supply to the tissues and help to increase the lymphatic drainage of waste products.

1 Soothe, warm and relax the thigh muscles with upward flowing effleurage strokes such as integration and fanning motions. Repeat several times, always returning the stroke to the back of the knee by gliding your hands around and down the sides of the leg.

2 Knead thoroughly over the whole area to enliven the thigh and buttock muscles and help the exchange of tissue fluids. Follow up with effleurage strokes to boost the circulation.

3 Deep friction strokes help to break up toxic deposits. Squeeze and rotate your thumb on one area at a time, using your other hand to push the tissue towards the stroke. Follow these strokes with fanning motions to aid the elimination process.

4 Pummel, hack and cup the thigh and buttocks, one hand following the other in rapid succession, flicking off the skin at the moment of contact.

5 Soothe the thighs and buttocks with effleurage strokes. If you have a mechanical roller, use it to add to the benefits of your cellulite massage by moving it in circular motions. This is particularly effective when the skin is oiled.

AROMATHERAPY IN PREGNANCY

Pregnancy can be one of the most exciting and fulfilling times of a woman's life. The joy of bringing another human being into the world creates a tremendous feeling of contentment and anticipation, but it is also a time of great physical and emotional upheaval. Together with the ever-important trio of exercise, good diet and rest, essential oils can play an important role in helping a woman cope with the stresses of pregnancy, the pain of labour and post-natal recovery.

RECOMMENDED ESSENTIAL OILS

Chamomile, geranium (in low doses), lavender, lemon, neroli, orange, rose, sandalwood.

For nausea:
Black pepper, ginger, lemon, nutmeg, rosewood, sandalwood.

To counteract heartburn:
Peppermint, lemon.

To combat fluid retention:
Geranium, grapefruit, mandarin, neroli, orange.

To tone the system in preparation for labour:
Geranium.

For lower back massage during labour:
Geranium, lemon, neroli.

For lower back massage in late pregnancy, blend 4 drops each lavender and sandalwood in 30 ml/2 tbsp carrier oil.

Spoil yourself with the luxurious and relaxing scent of rose for body and facial oils to keep your spirits up during pregnancy.

BLENDS AND REMEDIES FOR COMMON AILMENTS

Aromatherapy can help with many of the minor problems that may occur during pregnancy.

Heartburn
Avoid heavy meals and rich, spicy foods. Peppermint tea infusions help, or rub the solar plexus with a blend of 2 drops each lemon and peppermint in 15 ml/1 tbsp carrier oil.

Constipation
Make sure you eat plenty of fresh, high-fibre foods and drink plenty of still water. Tension can be a contributory factor, so try a relaxing bath with 3 drops lavender and 4 drops rose oil. Massage the abdomen and back with 4 drops chamomile or orange in 15 ml/1 tbsp carrier oil.

Sleep problems
A relaxing bath with 3 drops each neroli and rose will help you to get a good night's sleep, and you can add 2 drops ylang ylang for its calming, sedative effect. A couple of drops of rose or lavender on the pillow will help.

Sore breasts
These need extra care during pregnancy as they expand. Use gentle massage with 3 drops each rose and orange in 15 ml/1 tsbp sweet almond oil, or make a cool rose-water compress if your breasts are swollen. Sweet almond oil on its own is excellent for sore or cracked nipples during breast-feeding. Never use pure essential oils on the breasts during this period as they can easily be transferred to the baby during feeding.

Stretch marks
A daily massage around the hips and expanding tummy, using 2 drops mandarin and 1 drop neroli, or 5 drops lavender in 15 ml/1 tbsp jojoba, wheat germ or evening primrose oil, will help keep skin supple. Start around the fifth month and continue after the birth until you return to your normal weight.

Swollen ankles
Weight gain and fluid retention may result in swollen ankles. These can be reduced with a lukewarm footbath containing 2 drops each benzoin, rose and orange. Rest with feet raised whenever possible.

Varicose veins
Mix 2 drops each cypress, lemongrass and lavender into 30 ml/2 tbsp apricot kernel oil and smooth gently over the legs to give relief. If the veins are prominent, one of the best oils for the circulation is geranium, but this should always be very dilute for use during pregnancy. Add a maximum of 4 drops to the bath or to 15 ml/1 tbsp carrier oil to massage the leg with upward movements. Do not work directly over the veins or apply too much pressure.

EASING LOWER BACK STRAIN

Pregnancy can put a great deal of strain on the curvature of the lower spine and the surrounding muscles, sometimes leading to chronic back pain. Focus massage strokes on the lower back and buttocks, enabling the area to release its tension.

1 Spread oil over the lower back and buttocks, warming and soothing the muscles with soft effleurage strokes. Then begin to work deeper into the gluteal muscles of the buttocks, rotating the heel of the hand in one area at a time while supporting the hip with the other hand.

2 A pregnant woman will instinctively place a hand over the base of her spine to soothe away pain. Bring relief to the muscles surrounding and covering the pelvic girdle and lower back with flowing, circular motions from the surface of your hand.

3 Tiny, circular friction movements with the fingertips will deepen the remedial effects of strokes on the lower back. Ease away tension in the muscle that covers the sacrum, the flat triangular bone at the base of the spine, pushing the tissue towards the stroke with the other hand.

CIRCLING THE ABDOMEN

After the first three months of a healthy pregnancy, the abdomen can be gently massaged with soft circular movements. The warmth of your touch and the soporific motions will be very relaxing to both the mother and the baby.

LABOUR

To create a relaxing atmosphere, use a few drops of lavender in a vaporizer or try rose, neroli or ylang ylang to fortify you as time passes. If labour is progressing slowly, try marjoram in a massage oil or compress to stimulate contractions.

AFTER THE BIRTH

The "baby blues" often occur around the third or fourth day after birth, though some women can suffer a more severe form of post-natal depression for much longer. A bath with jasmine and ylang ylang will help you to feel better, or add a blend of chamomile, geranium and orange to a body oil to help with hormonal imbalance.

A bath with lavender will soothe perineal soreness. Add tea tree for its antiseptic properties.

CAUTIONS: The following oils should be avoided during pregnancy (particularly during the first five months) because of their strong diuretic properties, or tendency to induce menstruation: *bay, basil, clary sage, comfrey, fennel, hyssop, juniper, marjoram, melissa, myrrh, rosemary, thyme, sage.*

Use all essential oils in half the usual quantity during pregnancy and take extra care in handling them. Ensure that the oils you are using are pure essential oils, as adulterated blends or synthetic oils can sometimes have less predictable effects.

If you have a history of miscarriage you should also avoid chamomile and lavender for the first few months, although in general they are excellent oils for pregnancy.

Because of their potentially toxic nature and strong abortive qualities, the following oils should never be used except by a qualified aromatherapist, and must be avoided during pregnancy: *oreganum, pennyroyal, St John's wort, tansy, wormwood.*

BABY MASSAGE

All babies thrive on being cuddled, touched and massaged, for skin-to-skin contact is essential to the nurturing of a baby, helping her to bond with her parents and to develop emotional and physical health and self-esteem. Massage and touch can become a natural part of play with a young baby, especially during and after bath time, or before she is dressed. No formal routine is needed, just gently stroke the baby's body and limbs, using effleurage circles and fanning motions. Alternatively, softly squeeze, knead and perform passive movements on the arms, legs, fingers and toes. Your touch will comfort and soothe the baby, helping her to explore and discover the wonders of her body.

RECOMMENDED ESSENTIAL OILS

It is both safe and beneficial to use essential oils with babies and young children, as long as you ensure that the dosage is correctly prepared and you exercise common sense when selecting the oils. As a precaution, avoid the very stimulating, strong-smelling oils.

For newborn babies
For fretfulness:
Chamomile, geranium, lavender, mandarin.

For nappy rash and skin irritation:
Chamomile, lavender.

For cradle cap:
Eucalyptus (Eucalyptus radiata), geranium.

For teething:
Chamomile, lavender.
Dosage: 1–3 drops of essential oil in
30 ml/2 tbsp carrier oil.

For babies from 2–6 months
All the above oils are effective for babies of this age, as well as mandarin and neroli. For sickness, peppermint may be calming: put 1 drop on a cotton wool ball at the foot of the baby's cot.

CAUTION: Do not use peppermint for babies under 2 months. In cases of sickness you could try spearmint as an alternative.
Dosage: 3–5 drops of essential oil in
30 ml/2 tbsp carrier oil.

For babies from 6–12 months
In addition to the oils suggested above, grapefruit, palmarosa and tea tree can be used. For hyperactive children, essential oil of marjoram can be very helpful, but as this problem is usually complex it is important that you should seek the advice of your doctor as well.
Dosage: 3–5 drops of essential oil in
30 ml/2 tbsp carrier oil.

To alleviate the symptoms of coughs and colds in babies and children of all ages:
Eucalyptus, lavender and tea tree in a vaporizer.

SOOTHING AND FEATHERING

This routine will help the parent and baby form a loving, secure relationship.

1 Hold your baby close to you so she can feel the warmth of your body, the beat of your heart and the rhythm of your breathing, enabling her to melt into you and be comforted by your familiar presence.

2 Babies love to lie against the softness of your body. Soothe her by placing one hand over the base of her spine, while gently stroking her head.

3 Running your fingertips up and down the baby's back will make her giggle with pleasure as the featherlike touches brush her delicate skin.

EFFLEURAGE

If the baby can keep still for long enough, you can rub nourishing oil into her skin while giving her a massage. Soft effleurage strokes on her back, such as fanning and circles, will delight her.

KNEADING AND SQUEEZING

Chubby little arms and legs are made for gentle kneading and squeezing. Press the limbs softly between your thumb and fingers.

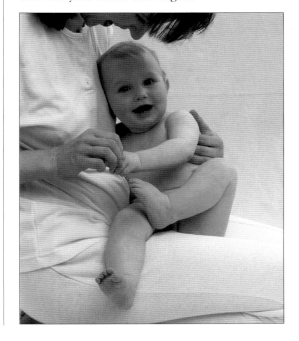

MASSAGE FOR THE ELDERLY

Many elderly people live full and active lives, and aromatherapy massage provides a valuable contribution to the maintenance of their physical and emotional health. The contact of touch through the medium of massage is especially important for alleviating feelings of isolation, which may result from loneliness or bereavement.

Using essential oils for the elderly presents no particular difficulties, but it is advisable to bear in mind two general points. First, as we age our metabolism slows down, so that any chemical introduced into the body will remain there slightly longer. Second, because of this slower metabolic rate and a less physically active life, the whole system can become more toxic. This is particularly true for those people who must necessarily live a more sedentary life through disability, or are in residential homes or hospitals.

It is best to avoid the highly stimulating oils and make use of those with gentler effects. A more dilute blend may also be advisable.

Whole body massage is beneficial to older people, but if they are uncomfortable about undressing, then massage on the hands, feet and face can also be helpful. Still, hands-on holds, to induce feelings of calm and peace, can be applied to the body just as well while the person is fully clothed.

Regular hand and footbaths with essential oils are an excellent preventive measure against stiff and aching joints in the extremities.

STILL HANDS-ON HOLDS

A condition commonly affecting the elderly is the onset of osteoarthritis, a degenerative disease of the joints caused by wear and tear. One or several joints of the body may be affected. Gentle massage with the recommended essential oils brings great relief. However, it is not advisable to massage over the joints if they are inflamed, swollen or disintegrated. In these circumstances, still holds will allow the warmth of your hands to subtly comfort the affected area, helping to increase circulation and reduce stiffness.

RECOMMENDED ESSENTIAL OILS

Frankincense, geranium, ginger, grapefruit, jasmine, juniper, lavender, marjoram, nutmeg, neroli, rosemary, sandalwood.

For arthritis:
Benzoin, black pepper, chamomile, cedarwood, eucalyptus, ginger, juniper, lemon, marjoram, nutmeg.

For aches and pains:
Ginger.

For grief and loneliness:
Marjoram, rose, nutmeg.

For constipation:
Black pepper, fennel, ginger, marjoram.

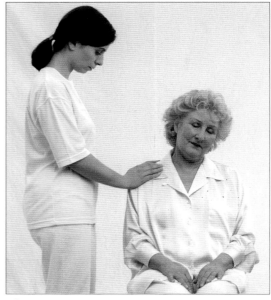

1 Focus your attention and breath into your hands before gently cradling the shoulder. This supportive hold will help the shoulder relax.

2 Osteoarthritis commonly affects the knee joints in older people. Cup the knee between your hands to bring it warmth and comfort.

RELAXING THE SPINE

Long periods of sitting still may cause tension and stiffness in the spine.

1 Soft, circular effleurage strokes over the top of the spine, at the base of the neck and between the shoulder blades, will ease away tension. While massaging with one hand, use the other hand to support the front of the body.

2 Excess tissue frequently builds up over stiff, tense areas, further inhibiting flexibility. Once the muscles are warmed with effleurage, sink into a deeper level of tissue with friction strokes. Use small circular motions from your fingertips to loosen and stretch the areas surrounding the top of the spine.

STAYING SUPPLE

Massaging the hands and feet will help to keep the wrists, fingers, ankles and toes supple, giving the whole system an extra boost.

1 Support the wrist with your fingers, and apply circular and sliding strokes with your thumbs to ease away tension from its tiny bones.

2 Many older people wish to pursue their hobbies, which may require dextrous hands and fingers. If the joints are not inflamed or degenerated, regular hand massage, with gentle passive movements and stretching of the fingers, will assist this continued flexibility in the hands.

A SOOTHING NECK AND FACE MASSAGE

This is an excellent way of easing away physical and emotional tension in elderly people. The loving contact of your hands is especially comforting in times of loneliness, distress or bereavement.

Support the head with a cushion or folded towel and apply gentle circular and sliding strokes with your fingertips to the neck and face working upwards to the hairline.

CONVALESCENCE AND RECUPERATION

After an illness or injury the body is left in a vulnerable condition, and a period of convalescence is vital to give the immune system time to rebuild its defences. Massage helps to promote this important transition from a period when the body is battling to heal itself to full recovery and a return to normal health.

The period of convalescence is usually a time of physical and emotional fluctuation. The patient may experience bursts of energy, followed by fatigue when the spirits fall. Gentle, hands-on holds are ideal for the first fragile stages of convalescence. The touch of your hands will comfort the body, stimulating the nerves that replenish the vital organs, and return the body to a normal resting state. As your partner recuperates, whole body massage will tone up the muscles, boosting circulation and increasing the body's overall vitality and sense of well-being.

RECOMMENDED ESSENTIAL OILS

To stimulate the appetite:
Black pepper, orange.

To overcome lethargy:
Black pepper, tea tree.

To comfort and lift the spirits:
Orange, nutmeg.

To boost the immune system:
Bergamot, black pepper, rosewood, tea tree.

Tonics: *Clary sage, mandarin.*

HEALING HOLDS

These soothing holds help to balance the nervous system and increase the body's energy levels. Your caring touch will stimulate the skin senses and help to restore emotional health and self-esteem, vital to the healing process. Start at the head, gently placing your hands over the forehead, temples and cheeks, then work methodically down both sides of the body to the feet. Proceed in a relaxed and unhurried manner, giving equal attention to all parts of the body.

2 Slowly withdraw your left hand and rest it on top of your right hand. Tune in to the heartbeat and the rise and fall of the breath.

1 Gently cup your left hand over your partner's temple and place your right hand over the heart area. This helps to encourage a sense of integration between mind and body.

3 Move to the side and rest one hand on the chest and one over the solar plexus. This helps to decrease anxiety and encourages deeper breathing.

CLEARING THE HEAD

A prolonged period of inactivity can cause the shoulder and neck muscles to tense up, restricting the circulation which, in turn, leads to headaches. Relax the shoulder and neck area by kneading the shoulders, then follow this with a neck, head and face massage.

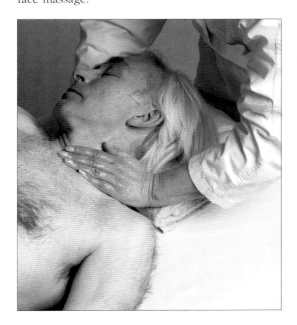

GETTING READY FOR ACTION

As your partner recuperates and becomes stronger, he will be eager to resume normal activities. When he has reached this stage in his convalescence, focus your massage on the feet and legs to boost a sluggish circulatory system, and massage the arms and hands to renew their strength and dexterity.

1 Massage the hands and fingers to release tension and increase flexibility. Use circular and sliding strokes with your thumbs and stretch the fingers gently.

2 Now massage the forearms, using draining strokes to help the circulation flow back to the heart. To loosen and warm the muscles, use one hand after the other in a fanning motion, working towards the elbow.

DEVELOPING YOUR KNOWLEDGE

Once you have become familiar with essential oils and with the practical benefits they offer, you may wish to gain
a deeper understanding of the nature of these aromatic substances.

M ost people begin to collect essential oils slowly, one by one, as they can afford them. You will usually choose oils to answer a particular need, or because you find a scent especially appealing. Having used the oils for a while you may become aware that your understanding of the use and benefits of a particular oil has deepened. This may become apparent with the realization that the aroma of the oil will relieve a painful or disquieting emotion or a physical symptom time after time. If you would like to explore this situation further, here are two exercises that may help.

ESSENTIAL OILS AND YOUR STATE OF MIND

The power essential oils possess to affect our state of mind is available to all of us if we actively choose to use them for one of these specific purposes. A suitable occasion might be prior to a very special social event, an interview or exam, or a period of study. You may also want to refresh yourself after an unpleasant experience such as an argument or an unwelcome visitor. The relaxing oils are helpful when preparing for meditation, or to clear the mind before going to sleep.

EXERCISE ONE

The first exercise uses the power of the imagination to take you on a journey inspired by an oil of your choice. You will need to choose a period of at least half an hour when you will not be interrupted. Find a comfortable upright chair, or a cushion on which you can sit comfortably on the floor; the essential oil of your choice, preferably one that you have used frequently for a reasonable period of time; and a handkerchief or paper tissue.

Put 1–2 drops of your chosen essential oil on to the handkerchief or tissue and place it within easy reach. Seat yourself comfortably. If you are sitting in a chair you may want to put a cushion under your feet to help you relax. Once you are in a comfortable position place your hands lightly, palms down, on your thighs. Concentrate on the rise and fall of your breath and become observant of your breath as it enters and leaves your body. If any thoughts of daily activities come into your head, acknowledge them and then allow them to pass away.

After a few minutes have passed, take the scented handkerchief and inhale from it deeply for one or two breaths. Try to observe which parts of the body you become aware of and what feelings are there – for example, it may be a warm sensation or a tingling one. Colours may come to mind, specific pictures, or perhaps a dream-like story. Allow the inspiration of the scent to transport you in your imagination, and as far as possible allow yourself really to trust what you imagine and feel. When the images begin to fade, gently bring your attention back to your own breathing, observing the rise and fall of your chest.

Become aware again of the comfortable chair in the room and, when you are completely ready, slowly open your eyes. You may feel a little dreamy after completing the exercise, and a glass

The stress that is often associated with periods of unusually hard work, or studying for an exam, may be eased by using an essential oil such as ginger or cedarwood.

of water or juice can help regain a solid, present feeling in your body. The activity of writing down any thoughts and feelings about the experience will also help achieve this.

By making this journey into the imagination several times with different essential oils it is possible to develop your confidence and intuitive knowledge. As a guide, the whole process should last approximately 15 minutes.

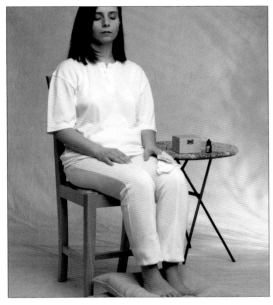

1 Choose a time when you will not be disturbed. Make sure you adopt a comfortable position, and put everyday concerns out of your mind.

2 When your mind is clear, take the handkerchief or tissue with the essential oil on it and inhale for one or two breaths.

EXERCISE TWO

The second exercise provides an alternative way of getting to know each essential oil in greater depth. You will need to have the bathroom to yourself for half an hour or more. You will also need the essential oil or oils of your choice, a candle securely fixed in a holder and some matches. Some people like to listen to a relaxing piece of music while bathing, so you may like to have this ready too.

Try to do this exercise at a time when you don't need to cleanse yourself thoroughly, so that the bath is purely relaxing. Run as deep a bath as you can, making sure the water is at a comfortable temperature. Meanwhile, blend the essential oils in a carrier oil.

When you are ready, concentrate on the purpose of the bath and light the candle. Put the blended essential oil into the bath just before you get into it. Remain in the bath for as long as you feel like it, or until the water is no longer comfortably warm. Allow any thoughts that float into your mind to come and go gently, and concentrate on any dreamlike images or colours inspired by the aromas rising in the steam.

This type of bath can be tremendously restorative as well as developing a heightened awareness of each of the oils you use in this way.

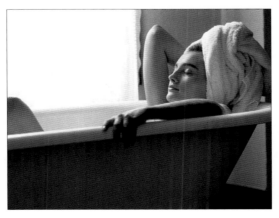

Enjoy your aromatherapy bath as a relaxation exercise rather than a cleansing routine, with plenty of time to absorb the aromas.

RECOMMENDED ESSENTIAL OILS

For a special occasion:
Clary sage, grapefruit, orange.

In preparation for an exam or interview:
Bergamot, black pepper, cedarwood, frankincense, ginger, grapefruit, lemon, neroli, orange, peppermint, rosemary, rosewood, sandalwood.

To help when studying:
Bergamot, eucalyptus, frankincense, ginger, grapefruit, jasmine, juniper, lemon, peppermint, rosemary, nutmeg.

For cleansing after difficult situations:
Cypress, eucalyptus, juniper, lavender, lemon, peppermint, rosemary.

To aid meditation:
Cedarwood, clary sage, frankincense, jasmine, palmarosa, rosewood, sandalwood.

Lighted candles or an aromatherapy burner, with the same oil as you have in the bath, will heighten the atmosphere.

MASSAGE

 The sense of touch is a powerful and highly sensitive form of communication. It is a natural reaction to reach out and touch, whether to feel the shape or texture of an object, or to respond to – perhaps to comfort – another person. A mother cuddles her baby, everyone strokes the family pets, loving partners caress, and if you accidentally bump into something, you instinctively rub the sore spot better.

To touch someone can mean different things in different cultures. There are many social restraints which inhibit touching in public. In western society, a formal handshake, a nod of the head or a peck on each cheek are all recognized forms of greeting, and can be carried out without any show of real emotion. This rather formal approach to physical contact is contrary to our most basic instincts and needs. Fortunately, we are now rediscovering the healing power of massage and other touch therapies, which have been understood in other cultures for thousands of years.

Massage is beneficial to the whole physiological system: it stimulates and warms the tissues, improves blood flow and the elimination of toxins, and soothes the nervous system by inducing a state of deep relaxation. It provides a safe and neutral situation in which to receive the loving touch that is so important for our emotional health and self-esteem.

THE ART OF MASSAGE

Massage can fairly claim to be the oldest form of healing in existence. The use of touch to relieve aching muscles, to give comfort or to express love is as old as humankind, and is something humans share with animals as an instinctive way of bonding and sharing. As a stress-reliever it is probably without equal, and every culture throughout history has used massage in some form: every language, ancient or modern, has a word for massage.

AN ANCIENT TRADITION

Written records mentioning massage date back some 5000 years. *The Yellow Emperor's Classic of Internal Medicine* advocated stroking the limbs to "protect against colds, keep the organs supple and prevent minor ailments". Ancient Sanskrit texts advocate the benefits of massage, and in India, the Ayurvedic scriptures, which are nearly 4000 years old, also recommend rubbing and shampooing the body to keep it healthy and to promote healing. The tradition of using massage has remained unbroken in India since that time: most mothers are taught to massage their newborn babies, and when they grow up the children are taught to massage their parents.

MASSAGE IN THE CLASSICAL WORLD

In ancient Greece the practice of rubbing up the limbs, or *anatripsis*, was highly recommended for treating fatigue, sports or battle injuries and illness. Hippocrates, the so-called "father" of medicine, writing in the fifth century BC, stated that the physician must be "experienced in many things but assuredly rubbing". He suggested that the way to health was to have a scented bath and an oiled massage every day. Greek medical centres, or

The Chinese have long believed in the therapeutic properties inherent in regular massage. Gentle manipulation of the limbs was said to have an improving effect on the circulation.

gymnasia, as they were known, nearly always included massage schools within them.

The Romans were equally enthusiastic about the benefits of massage, incorporating it into a daily routine in their spas alongside hot and cold baths; Julius Caesar had regular massages in an attempt to cure his epilepsy. The renowned Roman physician, Galen, wrote 16 manuals on the subject of massage, and introduced a variety of techniques and strokes that are still commonly used in massage today.

Massage continued to be popular and respected in Europe after the end of Roman

rule, although the elaborate Roman baths and massage facilities soon fell into disrepair. But with the rise of Christianity, the needs of the body came to be seen as self-indulgent and sinful, and massage was neglected.

THE FOUNDATIONS OF MODERN MASSAGE

From the time of the Renaissance, when classical medicine and philosophy were once again in favour, massage was revived and respected once more. In 14th-century France, the physician Guy de Chauliac wrote a classic textbook in which he promoted hands-on techniques of manipulation as being highly complementary to surgical science.

Massage strokes were often recommended as cures for common ailments in the late 19th century.

With the spread of the Ottoman Empire came Turkish-style bath and massage treatments. As the benefits of regular body work were recognized, massage became a firmly established part of beauty rituals for the wealthy.

The foundations of modern massage and physiotherapy are based on a system devised by the Swede, Per Henrik Ling (1776–1839). Ling studied the human body in activity and at rest, and developed a system of medical gymnastics, exercises and massage, based upon ancient techniques learned while travelling through China. His research led to a royal appointment and the formation of an institute of massage. Ling's classification of strokes forms the basis of modern western massage.

HOLISTIC MASSAGE

Holistic massage, as described in this book, is the most popular of recent developments in massage. Recognizing the mind, body and spirit connection, holistic therapy looks at releasing trapped emotional issues and creating overall health and balance, rather than simply easing tired muscles and aching limbs.

The return to the premise that the caring touch is itself a powerful agent makes holistic massage suitable for a varied list of treatments. The massage uses the basic strokes of Swedish massage but works more gently, with the emphasis on relaxing the client psychologically and emotionally, as well as physically. The focus on relaxation applies to the practitioner as well, so that the experience has a calm and meditative quality for both people. The strokes remain important to the treatment, but it is the caring and loving quality of the touch that is fundamental to the holistic principle.

THE EFFECTS OF MASSAGE

When applied with skill and care, massage can evoke many beneficial changes within the body, mind and spirit. While the strokes ease pain and tension from stiff and aching muscles, boost a sluggish circulation or eliminate toxins, the nurturing touch of the hands soothes away mental stress and restores emotional equilibrium.

THE IMPORTANCE OF TOUCH

Massage provides a safe and neutral situation in which to receive the caring touch, which is so important for emotional health and self-esteem. Touch is fundamental to the development of a healthy human being, but the need to be touched does not stop with the end of childhood. Unfortunately, in many societies, physical contact between adults is strictly limited to intimate relationships.

The loving touch of massage unlocks not only the physical tensions trapped in muscles, but also acknowledges, with complete acceptance, the essence of the person within. While the massage itself is active, the underlying quality of the touch is one of stillness and calm, at one with the person receiving it. This is why massage is so beneficial; it helps you to feel safe enough to relax and unwind from the deepest parts of your mind.

REDUCING STRESS

Massage allows time for the replenishment of innate resources of vital energy. This is particularly relevant in the modern world when stress is known to be the root cause of many serious physical and mental conditions. Stress is a natural factor of life, but if it is not discharged appropriately, or is prolonged unduly, it robs the body of health and energy.

The power of touch easily transcends more formal means of communication as a pathway to deeper relaxation, increased vitality and greater self-awareness, to the benefit of both body and soul.

Stress can also lower the natural defences of the immune system. If you are constantly exposed to the adverse effects of stress, it can lead to anxiety, depression, lethargy, insomnia and panic attacks. Massage is increasingly recognized as a successful treatment for the symptoms arising from stress.

PHYSIOLOGICAL BENEFITS

Massage can both stimulate and relax the body. The skin, blood and lymphatic systems are all stimulated, boosting circulation, aiding cellular renewal and removing toxic waste. As tense muscles relax, stiff joints loosen and nerves are soothed, and an all-over feeling of relaxation and well-being is induced.

The nervous system

The nervous system is a highly complex network which relays messages from the brain to the rest of the body. The part of the nervous system that regulates many physiological functions leaves the brain at the base of the skull and runs down the spinal cord, protected by the spine's bony vertebrae. Depending on the depth of the movements used, the nerve endings can be stimulated or soothed in massage.

The skin

With massage comes an increase in blood circulation. This helps the exfoliation of superficial dead skin cells, tones the skin and encourages its renewal process. Massage helps to maintain the collagen fibres, which give skin its elasticity and strength and keep wrinkles at bay. The activity of the sweat and sebaceous glands, which lubricate and moisturize the skin, is regulated.

Muscles

With the increase in blood flow, the blood's vital nutrients circulate more efficiently. Massage is popular with sportspeople because it can improve muscle tone, restore mobility and ensure the elimination of waste products after exercise. Regular massage helps strains and sprains to heal more rapidly, and relaxes calf cramps and stiff muscles. Massage before an exercise session will help loosen and warm up the muscles; afterwards it will ease sore and aching limbs.

Circulation and lymphatic systems

By dilating the blood vessels, massage helps to increase the blood circulation, vital for the healthy functioning of the whole body.

At the same time, improved blood circulation helps accelerate the lymphatic system, which absorbs and eliminates waste products. Massage is an important way of speeding up the flow of lymph, thus providing the body with a strong immune system to fight against infections and disease.

The digestive system

Massage mobilizes the digestive system, helping problems such as constipation and flatulence. The digestive system is quick to respond to stress, and the reduction in tension that comes with regular massage has a regulating effect on the digestion.

A calm and meditative environment contributes greatly to the therapeutic effect of a massage. Let go of any mental tensions before you begin as these can compromise the mood you are creating.

Placing your hands on the body of someone else can be one of the most direct ways to make contact with their inner being and help them to relax.

Massage allows an opportunity to connect with the energy of another person, and this in turn will help to increase your own sensitivity.

MASSAGE OILS

Throughout the world, people giving massage use locally available oils, usually vegetable oils, to help the hands flow and glide over the skin. Olive oil, goose grease, goat butter and other lubricants have all been used at times; in parts of Africa a handful of oily dough is used to absorb dirt and toxins from the skin surface as the massage soothes the muscles.

Some oils are more pleasant and versatile than others, and have a beneficial effect on the skin in themselves. Probably the most useful oil, and the one most widely used in professional massage, is sweet almond oil. It is light, non-greasy and easily absorbed by the skin. Neutral and non-allergenic, it is even suitable for massaging babies. Grapeseed oil seems to suit oily skins quite well; it is reasonably priced and widely available. Rather thicker, but still a useful alternative, is soya oil.

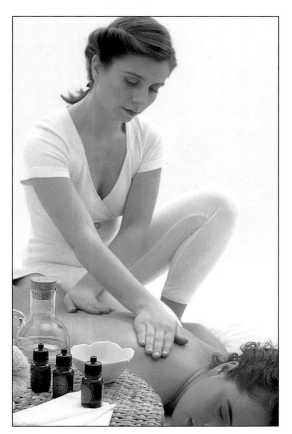

Sunflower oil may be used for massage if nothing else is available, though it may give a slight hint of salad dressing! Olive oil certainly does, although this was traditionally used in Mediterranean countries. Do not use mineral oils, such as baby oil: they sit on the surface of the skin and feel very greasy.

ENRICHING THE OIL BLEND

Other oils extracted from nuts or seeds all have their own particular qualities and, while they may be a little sticky and rich to use on their own for massage, they can be added to a lighter vegetable oil to create a mixture especially suitable for an individual skin type.

Walnut oil acts as a co-ordinator and balances the nervous system; like evening primrose oil, it can help to alleviate menstrual problems, including pre-menstrual tension. Sesame oil is ideal for stretch marks. Apricot kernel, peachnut and evening primrose oils are all good for cell regeneration and are particularly useful for face massage. Hazelnut oil is astringent and therefore good for oily skin, while jojoba benefits oily and sensitive skins and is valuable in the treatment of acne. For dry skins, a little wheat germ oil or avocado oil may be added.

These oils are all rich in nutrients, but when buying them, check that they have been naturally processed and not chemically treated. Cold-pressed oils are always the best.

Essential oils, blended into the base oil, will enhance the therapeutic effect of the whole massage experience with their own special properties and fragrance.

ESSENTIAL OILS

Essential oils may be added to the base oils, both for fragrance and for their therapeutic effects. By spreading evenly and easily over the skin, the massage oils encourage the quick absorption of the therapeutic oils into the skin.

Essential oils are highly concentrated and should be treated with respect: if in doubt, do not use them, and if any skin irritation occurs, wash the oil off immediately with warm water and a mild soap.

Always buy essential oils in dropper bottles, and dilute them safely for use on the skin. As a general rule, up to 5 drops of essential oil in 10 ml/2 tsp carrier oil is enough for a body massage. Never be tempted to use more essential oil than the amount recommended.

Store essential oils in their dropper bottles, in a cool, dry place and away from inquisitive children.

CAUTIONS: Essential oils are wonderful natural remedies for a variety of problems, and their aromatic effects can enhance mood, release tensions and reduce stress. But they are highly concentrated substances and must be used with caution. Follow the points listed below and, for the treatment of persistent problems, always ask the advice of a qualified aromatherapist. If in *any* doubt at all, seek a medical opinion before using essential oils.

• Never take essential oils internally, unless professionally prescribed.

• Do not use the same oils for more than one or two weeks at any one time in the treatment of specific ailments.

• When mixing your own blends, do not use more than three oils in any one treatment as the synergistic effects are less predictable.

• Do not use oils in pregnancy without first getting professional advice. The following oils are strongly contra-indicated at this time: bay, basil, cedarwood, clary sage, comfrey, fennel, hyssop, juniper, marjoram, melissa, myrrh, rosemary, sage and thyme.

• For anyone who has skin problems, test the diluted oil on a small area first. Dilute the oils even more than recommended, and if any skin irritation occurs, stop using the oils immediately. Do not use wheat germ oil on anyone who has an allergy to wheat. A few essential oils, such as bergamot, make the skin more sensitive to sunlight, and should be used with caution in hot, sunny weather.

• Be extra careful with anyone who has asthma or epilepsy. If they do experience a reaction, wash the oil off immediately.

MIXING OILS FOR MASSAGE

1 Assemble all the ingredients for your blend, but keep the essential oils covered until needed. Measure out your chosen base oil into a bowl.

2 Add a small amount of a richer vegetable oil if you wish to make a blend to suit a particular skin type. Add the essential oil, one drop at a time, and mix gently to blend. Keep the oil covered during the massage to minimize evaporation of the essential oil.

Adding an appropriate essential oil can heighten the effect of a massage considerably.

RECOMMENDED OIL BLENDS

For a generally relaxing massage blend, try essential oils of lavender and marjoram in equal amounts in a base vegetable oil. Both of these help to release tense, tired muscles and to induce a warm, relaxed glow. For a more invigorating, uplifting blend, add essential oils of bergamot and geranium to your massage oil. These have a refreshing effect on the whole system.

CHOOSING ESSENTIAL OILS

Essential oils may be extracted from exotic plants such as sandalwood or ylang ylang, or from more common plants like lavender and chamomile, but each one has its own characteristics and properties. The power of aromatics is quite subtle – as you get to know the different oils, you will come to understand their effects and learn which ones will blend well together. Never try to sniff a pure essential oil straight from the bottle, but place a single drop on the side of a glass.

Bergamot *(Citrus bergamia)*

This is the most effective antidepressant of all, best used at the start of the day. Do not use before going into bright sunlight, as it increases photosensitivity.

Bergamot

Black pepper *(Piper nigrum)*

The essential oil of black pepper is warming, comforting and sweet. It is very effective for poor circulation, aches and pains and stiffness.

Cedarwood *(Cedrus atlantica)*

The sweet, woody aroma of cedarwood oil has a calming effect. Use for skin complaints such as acne, alopecia, dandruff and eczema.

Chamomile *(Anthemis nobilis)*

Chamomile is relaxing and antispasmodic, helping to relieve tension headaches, nervous digestive problems and insomnia. It is also for useful and menstrual and menopausal problems.

Cypress *(Cupressus sempervirens)*

Astringent and antispasmodic, cypress can be used for circulatory problems, colds and coughs, menstrual problems and nervous tension. Do not use on anyone who suffers from high blood pressure.

Eucalyptus *(Eucalyptus globulus)*

One of the finest oils for respiratory complaints. Well diluted (never use more than 1 drop to 5 ml/ 1 tsp base oil), it can be applied to the forehead to relieve a hot, tense headache linked with tiredness. It has a cooling effect, reduces fever and is also a remedy for muscular or rheumatic aches and pains.

Geranium *(Pelargonium graveolens)*

The rose-scented geranium has useful properties, including its ability to bring a blend together for a more harmonious scent. Geranium has a refreshing, antidepressant quality, good for nervous tension, exhaustion, circulatory and skin problems.

Geranium

Ginger *(Zingiber officinale)*

The essential oil of ginger is known for its balancing nature. It is helpful in cases of muscular aches and pains, poor circulation, coughs and colds, rheumatism, nausea and loss of appetite. The oil is comforting and grounding at the same time; it

Ginger

can warm flat and cold emotions, and will sharpen the senses and memory. It blends well with citrus oils, neroli, rose and sandalwood, but should be used only in the lowest concentrations.

Jasmine *(Jasminum officinale)*

A favourite of the Arabs, Indians and Chinese, jasmine has a relaxing, euphoric effect. It can greatly lift the mood when there is debility, depression and listlessness. It will relieve menstrual cramps and is soothing to inflamed or irritated skin.

Juniper *(Juniperus communis)*

Juniper's most important use is as a detoxifier; it is effective for cellulite and in cases such as an absence of menstrual periods, cystitis, water retention and painful periods. Juniper should be avoided by people with kidney disease. It is uplifting and warming, and is known to be a helpful aid in coping with challenging situations.

Lavender *(Lavandula angustifolia/officinalis)*

One of the safest and most versatile of all essential oils, lavender has been used for centuries as a

Lavender

refreshing fragrance and as a remedy for stress-related ailments. It is especially helpful for tension headaches or for nervous digestive upsets. Use in a blend for a deeply relaxing and calming experience.

Lemon (Citrus limonum)

Possibly the most cleansing and antiseptic of the citrus oils, lemon is useful for boosting the immune system and in skin care, when it is effective on oily skin. It can also refresh and clarify the thoughts. Like all citrus oils, it deteriorates quickly.

Marjoram (Origanum majorana)

Marjoram has a calming, warming effect, and is good for both cold, tight muscles and for tense people who suffer from anxiety headaches, migraines and insomnia. Use in massage blends for rubbing into tired and aching muscles, especially in the evening to encourage a good night's sleep. It blends well with bergamot, lavender and rosemary.

Neroli (Citrus aurantium)

Neroli is one of the finest of the floral essences. Its effect is uplifting and calming, bringing a feeling of

Marjoram

peace. It is useful during times of anxiety, panic, hysteria, shock and fear. It can help promote self-esteem and is particularly effective for nervous diarrhoea and other stress-related conditions.

Orange (Citrus aurantium)

Refreshing but sedative, orange is a tonic for anxiety and depression, having a similar effect to neroli, distilled from the blossom of the same plant. Orange also stimulates the digestive system and is effective for constipation. Because the oil oxidizes very quickly, it cannot be kept for very long.

Palmarosa (Cymbopogon martini)

Palmarosa was used to adulterate the highly prized rose oil known as attar of roses, gaining the name "Indian" or "Turkish" oil. This refreshing oil is gentle and comforting, and effective for skin inflammations, scars, weak digestion and headaches.

Peppermint

Peppermint (Mentha piperita)

Peppermint's analgesic and antispasmodic effects make it very useful for muscular aches and pains, sore feet, indigestion and flatulence, stomach cramps, nausea, colds and fevers. Diluted in a base oil, it can be rubbed on to the temples to ease tension headaches.

Rose (Rosa x damascena trigintipetala)

The scent evokes a general sense of pleasure and happiness. The actions of the oil are sedating, calming and anti-inflammatory. Not surprisingly, rose oil has a wide reputation as an aphrodisiac, and where anxiety is a factor it can be very beneficial. Add to a base massage oil to soothe muscular and nervous tension. It is particularly good for older, drier skins.

Rose

Rosemary (Rosmarinus officinalis)

With a very penetrating, stimulating aroma, rosemary has been used for centuries to help relieve nervous exhaustion, tension headaches and migraines. Rosemary stimulates the lymphatic system, improves circulation to the brain, and is an excellent oil for mental fatigue and debility. Avoid in cases of high blood pressure.

Sandalwood (Santalum album)

Probably the oldest perfume in history, sandalwood is known to have been used for over 4000 years. It has a relaxing, antidepressant effect on the nervous system, and where depression causes sexual problems, sandalwood can be a genuine aphrodisiac. Massage enhances its soothing effects.

Tea tree (Melaleuca alternifolia)

Tea tree oil is active against all types of infectious organisms; it is also a very powerful immune stimulant, increasing the body's ability to respond to these organisms. Its effect is cooling and refreshing, helping to clear the head. Vigorous and revitalizing, it is particularly useful after shock.

Ylang ylang (Cananga odorata)

This intensely sweet essential oil has a sedative yet antidepressant action. It is good for many symptoms of excessive tension, such as insomnia, panic attacks, anxiety and depression. It also has a good reputation as an aphrodisiac, through its ability to reduce stress levels. It blends well with bergamot, sandalwood and jasmine.

PREPARING FOR MASSAGE

Creating the right environment and space for treatment can contribute to making massage an even more relaxing and beneficial experience. Knowing that you are carefully prepared and in control will help your massage partner to relax completely. Your own state of mind is important, too, so take the time to compose yourself before you begin.

PREPARING THE ROOM

Before you start, make sure that the room is pleasantly warm and draught-free, and choose a quiet time when you will not be disturbed. If you are going to give the massage on the floor, pad the area with a thick layer of blankets or towels, or use a futon, so that your partner will be truly comfortable. It is not a good idea to massage on a bed, as the give of the mattress will counteract much of your effort.

Have plenty of freshly laundered towels ready to cover areas of the body that are not being worked on. If you are using oil, place it in a convenient spot where you can reach it easily without the risk of knocking it over.

PREPARING YOURSELF

Wear loose-fitting clothes for massage, ideally short-sleeved, with soft-soled, flat shoes, or work in bare feet. Take off your watch and any rings or bracelets, and make sure your nails are short. Take time to compose yourself so that your whole attention is focused on the massage. Try to do a few stretches and take some deep breaths to help you to feel calm; if you give a massage when you are tense yourself, this may be transmitted to your massage partner. This can work the other way round too, so feel prepared mentally to let go of any tensions that you feel coming from the other person's body and avoid absorbing these stresses yourself.

Give your partner privacy to undress, and clear directions on how to lie down on the mattress. Use the towels correctly to cover your partner's body. As well as keeping warm, a sense of modesty may be crucial to your partner's relaxation, and by following these suggestions, you will immediately make them feel safe and secure in your hands.

Freshly laundered towels, soft cushions and fragrant oils will all add to the comfort of your partner.

Instruments can play a useful role in self-massage.

MAKING CONTACT

Establish contact with your partner by placing your hands gently down on to the body, so that one hand rests on the top of the spine and the other at its base. Check that your own body is relaxed while giving your partner a few moments to settle into a comfortable position. When using oil, pour it on to your own hands first to warm it, never directly on to your partner's skin, as cold oil can cause an unpleasant shock – undoing the relaxing effect. Using smooth, flowing strokes, spread the oil slowly on to the skin, then begin the massage.

Make sure you have to hand everything you will need in the course of the massage, including a plentiful supply of tissues and the chosen oils.

Candles and soft lighting will help create a mellow atmosphere and encourage relaxation.

Making the initial contact is a key moment in the massage. The calm, unhurried way that you first touch your partner can lay the foundation for a soothing, unwinding experience.

BASIC STROKES

When many people think of massage they picture the vigorous pummelling and slapping often associated with puritanical health spas. In truth, firm massage can be highly beneficial without causing discomfort. Alternate firm and gentle flowing strokes to create a combination that will alleviate tension and muscular aches and pains while invigorating the body. There are four basic types of movement in Swedish massage: effleurage, petrissage, friction and tapotement.

EFFLEURAGE

Effleurage describes long, soothing, stroking movements, using the flat of the hand (or fingers if you are working on small areas). These strokes are often used to apply oil. You can use one hand on its own or with the other providing support on top of it, both hands at once or each hand alternately.

Effleurage is used to start off a massage, soothing the nerve endings and helping your partner to get used to your touch. It is used again at the end for a relaxing finish. In between, effleurage movements provide an important link between other, more stimulating strokes and are used to make first contact with a new area of the body. If you ever feel hesitant about what to do next, insert a few effleurage strokes to maintain continuity.

Repeat effleurage strokes several times. Each time, try to start the first complete stroke with light pressure, then apply slightly more pressure with the next complete stroke. Where there are large muscle areas, such as the thighs and back, you can apply the most pressure for a more stimulating effect.

Relax the hands and mould them to the body. Use slow, continuous movements and keep your hands in contact with your partner between strokes.

CIRCLING

A movement allied to effleurage is circling, where the hands move large areas of muscle in a circular motion. Tension within muscles can produce knotted areas that may need working along or across the length of the fibres; this circular action starts to release the knots before deeper movements are used. It is essentially a slow, relaxing type of movement and should not be rushed.

1 Lay both hands parallel to each other and flat on the area you intend to massage, keeping them about 10 cm/4 in apart. Circle both hands clockwise.

2 Lift up the right hand as it completes the first half-circle to allow the left hand to pass underneath it in an unbroken motion.

3 As the left hand continues to circle over the body, cross the right hand over it, dropping it lightly back on to the skin.

4 Let the right hand form another half-circle stroke before lifting off as the left hand completes its full circle. Repeat the sequence several times.

PETRISSAGE

A number of massage movements involve various ways of kneading, rolling and picking up the skin and muscles. These movements firm and strengthen the structures by stimulating the deep layers of tissue, increasing the supply of blood to the area and improving the flow of lymph. Generally, a single group of muscles, or an individual muscle, is worked on at one time. The basic kneading action is similar to kneading dough. With light kneading you are tackling the top muscle layers, while firmer kneading works further down, easing taut muscles and freeing congested tissues to eliminate waste products.

All muscular activity produces potentially toxic waste materials, notably lactic acid. If the person also gets tense and stiff, these wastes are trapped within the muscles, making them ache even more. Petrissage is a very effective way of encouraging the drainage of lactic acid and other waste matter, which in turn allows new blood to flow in, bringing oxygen and fresh nutrients to each cell.

For petrissage, or kneading, start with your fingers pointing away from you, press down with your palm, grasp the flesh between fingers and thumb and push it towards the other hand. As you release the first hand your second hand grasps the flesh and pushes it back towards the first hand. It is a continuous action, alternating the hands to squeeze and release.

WRINGING

Another important petrissage-type movement is wringing, where the action of one hand against the other creates a powerful squeezing action in the muscles. When performed on the back, the person's own spine acts as a block against which the muscles are wrung. Make sure that your hands reach right round both sides of the body with each stroke, in order to get the most from the movement. Increase the speed of the stroke for an invigorating effect, then slow down towards the end for a soothing finish.

1 Place your right hand over the hip opposite to you and cup your left hand over the hip closest to you. Slide your hands towards each other with enough pressure to lift and roll the flesh on the sides of the body.

2 Decrease the pressure as you stroke across the back, hands passing each other to the opposite sides of the body. Without stopping, immediately begin to slide them back. Stroke your hands back and forth continuously while you wring up and down the lower back.

FRICTION

Friction, or "connective tissue massage", is a penetrating circular movement which applies direct pressure to a particular site of muscular tension, using the thumb, fingertips or knuckles. It is a valuable technique for concentrating on specific areas of tightness and muscle spasm in the back.

In general, pressure techniques are less painful when performed along the direction of the muscle fibres, rather than across them. Pressure is achieved by steadily leaning into the movement with the whole body, not by tensing your hands. The depth of the pressure applied should be adjusted for individual comfort; thinner people usually need lighter pressure and vice versa.

CAUTION: Do not attempt deep work if you are at all unsure of the effect, or if any pain occurs. Underdo rather than overdo the massage – effleurage and petrissage movements on their own can make a complete and thoroughly relaxing massage.

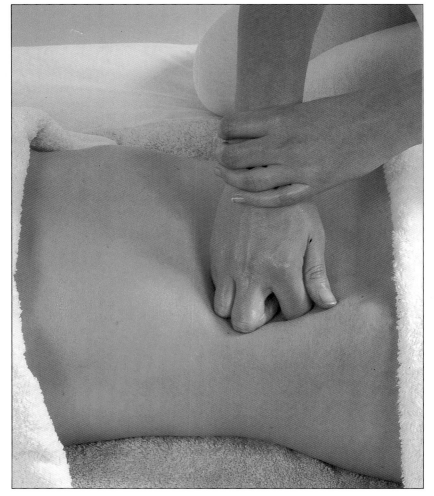

As you make the circular rotations you should actually feel the underlying tissues moving; you are not simply sliding over the surface of the skin. A variation on circular friction is static pressure, where you lean gradually into the muscle, slowly deepening the pressure without the rotation action. Press for a few seconds, then gradually release.

Another friction movement is knuckling: use the knuckles in a loosely clenched fist to produce rippling, circular motions. This movement is used to release tension up the sides of the spine and in other areas. Remember not to work directly over the spinal bone.

TAPOTEMENT

Tapotement, or percussion movements, are fast and stimulating. They include cupping, pummelling and hacking, which all sound like painful practices but which, when carried out properly, should certainly not cause bruising or pain. For all these movements, remember to keep your hands and wrists relaxed. All the percussion techniques are fast, precision actions, bringing one hand quickly after the other into contact with your partner. It is particularly important to ask your partner at the beginning whether you are applying the right degree of pressure.

These sequences stimulate the blood circulation, and also tone and help to strengthen sagging skin and muscles. In particular, they can tighten up areas of soft tissue, such as thighs and buttocks, which are prone to cellulite. Intersperse these brisk movements with gentler effleurage strokes.

CAUTION: Do not use percussion movements on particularly bony areas of the body as they will cause discomfort. As with all massage movements, never apply pressure on or below broken or varicose veins, only on the part of the leg which is higher than the vein (that is, closer to the heart).

For cupping, gently curve the hands to make a loose cupped shape, bending at the knuckles while keeping the fingers firmly together. Do not bend the fingers too far over. Using the cupped palm, make a bouncy, brisk, cupping action against a fleshy area, alternating the hands quickly. The fast action creates a suction against the skin. Try this movement on the back, buttocks and thighs.

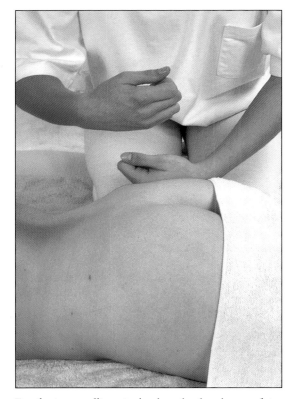

For the pummelling stroke, loosely clench your fists, but keep the wrists relaxed. You can make the strokes in two ways: either striking your partner with the outer edges of the loose fists, or with the front of the knuckles. Either way, the speed and rhythm of the movement is similar: brisk and firm, alternating the hands, without thumping your partner too enthusiastically. Once again, keep to the fleshier parts of the body, particularly cellulite zones such as hips, buttocks and thighs.

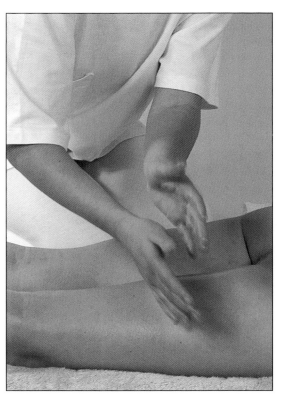

In hacking, the outer edge of the hand is used to stimulate the area by striking it quickly with alternate hands. You need to practise a brisk, bouncing movement, working rhythmically and rapidly over a fleshy area of the body. You need to have very relaxed wrists and fingers, and use the sides of the palm rather than the fingers. Used over the buttocks and thighs, hacking will help to tone up muscle and disperse excess fluid.

ELF-MASSAGE

One of the nicest things about massage is that you do not need to invest in expensive equipment to perform the movements, and indeed several strokes can also be successfully used for self-massage. The advantage of working on your own muscles is that you will know exactly how deeply you can press, getting instant feedback from your body about the effects of the massage. Another benefit is that it helps you to practise the techniques and gain confidence before applying them to a partner. Obviously, it is not possible to do a complete massage on yourself, and therapeutically it cannot equal the experience of relaxing on a couch and surrendering yourself to an expert massage treatment. However, you will find that there are many times when you can help yourself if your body calls out for some physical work to relieve aching muscles.

Many activities inevitably lead to tensions in some part of the body, and regular quick massages can help both to ease these tensions and to prevent more chronic aches and pains. At any time of the day a short self-massage can help you to feel revitalized and reduce the impact of stress, both physical and mental. Follow these simple techniques whenever you are feeling stiff, aching or jaded, to de-stress your system and to help yourself look and feel better.

SHOULDERS

The build-up of tension and pain in the neck and shoulders are common symptoms of today's pressured and stressful work environments. Wherever you are, you can unknot tense muscles with these simple techniques.

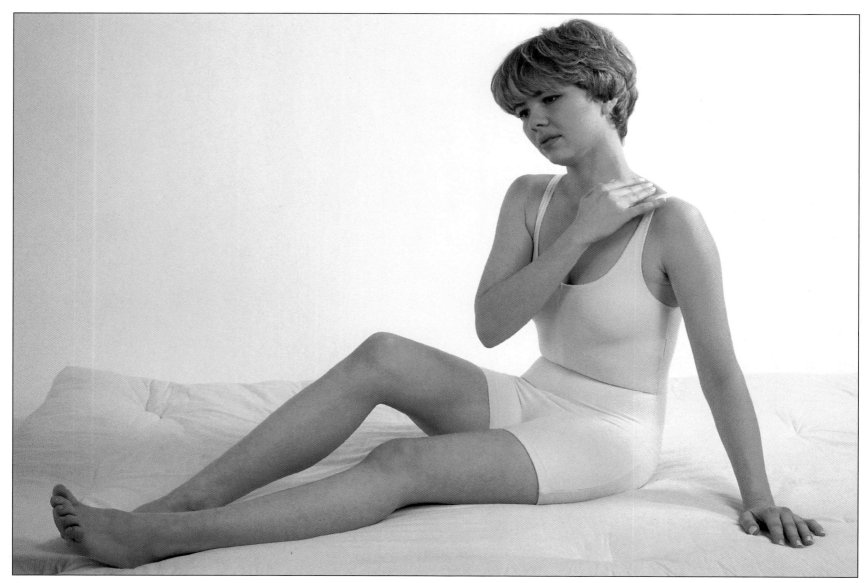

1 Sitting upright, start from the base of the neck and press down with your fingers along the top of the shoulders. As you reach the bony part of the shoulder, slide your hand back to the base of the neck, and repeat the pressing at least three times. Finish by stroking firmly from neck to shoulder and then repeat on the other side of the neck.

2 Use the fingertips of both hands to make small circular movements, working up the back of the neck. Gentle circular movements, where you can feel yourself easing muscular tightness, are better than direct, static pressures on this area. Continue up and round the base of the skull.

Peppermint essential oil works well for everyday aches and pains.

3 Knead each shoulder with a firm squeezing action, rolling the flesh between your fingers and the ball of your hand. Repeat several times on each side.

4 With your hand in a loose fist, pummel your shoulder lightly, keeping the wrist and elbow relaxed. Use light, springy movements to stimulate the area. Repeat on the other shoulder.

ARMS AND HANDS

Muscular tension forms in the arms and hands for a number of reasons. It may be a result of poor posture causing the shoulders to stiffen and leading to inflexibility in the arms, or may stem from repetitive movements at work which put strain on the muscles and tendons. Arm and hand massage is both relaxing and revitalizing.

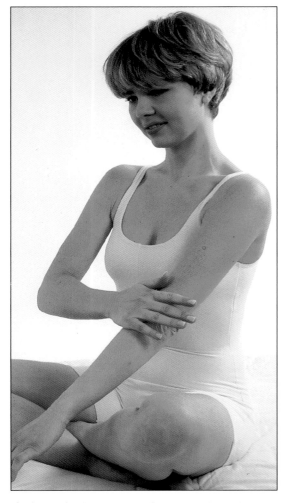

1 Stroke firmly up the arm from the wrist to the shoulder, returning with a lighter touch. Repeat the stroke several times on different parts of the arm.

2 Pressing your fingers towards the palm of the hand, knead up the arm from the elbow to the shoulder. Cover the area thoroughly, working right around the arm.

4 With thumb and fingers, make circular pressures around the elbow. First, work around the far side of the elbow with your working arm coming over the top of the arm you are massaging, then bend that arm up and work from the inside of your elbow. You may need to apply more oil for dry elbows.

3 Starting from the wrist, knead up the forearm towards the elbow, this time using your thumb to make circular movements.

5 Gently but briskly pat your upper arm, or use some gentle cupping. Finish with some effleurage stroking up and down the whole arm again.

6 Squeeze the hand firmly, spreading the palm laterally. Cover the whole of the hand, fingers and wrist in this way.

7 Using circular pressure, squeeze each finger joint between your finger and thumb. Then hold the base of each finger and pull the finger gently to stretch it, sliding your grip up to the top of the finger in one continuous movement.

8 With circular thumb pressures, work up each of the furrows between the bones in the hand from the knuckle to the wrist. When you have covered each furrow, smooth the hand by stroking.

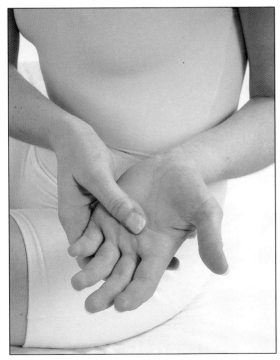

9 Turn the hand over to work on the palm. Cover the area with circular thumb pressures, paying particular attention to the heel of the hand and the wrist. Follow this with some deeper static pressures all over the palm.

10 Finish by stroking the palm of one hand with the other. This can be quite a firm stroke, working from the tips of the fingers to the wrist, leading with the pressure from the heel of the hand. Stroke back to the fingers and repeat twice more, each time using slightly less pressure. Finally, stroke the inside of the wrist. Repeat the whole sequence on the other arm and hand.

BACK AND ABDOMEN

Incorrect posture, long periods of standing or lifting heavy weights can all lead to pain in the lower back, while tension in the abdomen often reflects emotional unease and bottled-up feelings. A skilled, sensitive massage is the answer to both problems, but in the short term you may be able to relieve the discomfort a little with these techniques.

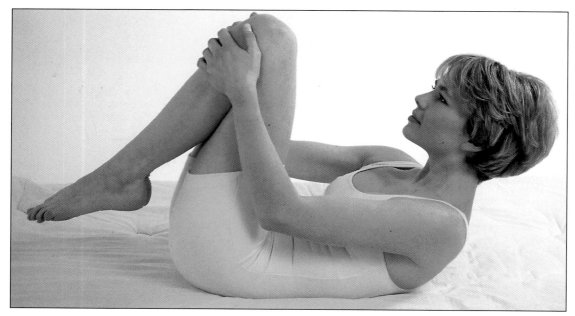

1 Lie on your back on the floor, clasp your knees and gently rock yourself backwards and forwards to massage the lower back, buttocks and hip joints, and gently stretch out the vertebrae.

2 Bend your knees up and use some gentle petrissage to knead the whole of the abdominal area. When you have finished kneading, place both hands flat on the centre of the abdomen, fingers pointing slightly together, and pause for a few moments. Then smooth your hands outwards over the hips and thighs in one long, slow, moulding movement.

BUTTOCKS, HIPS AND THIGHS

If you have an accumulation of cellulite in these areas, a quick daily massage using percussion and kneading movements will help to shift fatty deposits under the skin.

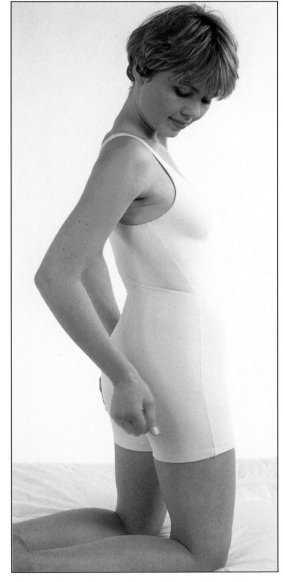

1 Kneel up and pummel your hips and buttocks, using a clenched fist. Keep your wrists flexible.

2 With the thumb and fingers, squeeze and release the muscles firmly and slowly, working from the top of the thigh over the buttock. Repeat the same movements on the other side.

3 Use both hands to squeeze and release the muscles on the front and side of the thigh, kneading the entire upper leg. Repeat on the other side.

4 Starting at the knee, stroke up the thigh with both hands to soothe the leg.

The essential oil of ginger will boost a sluggish circulation and help in the fight against cellulite.

LEGS AND FEET

Stroking and kneading movements will warm and stretch the large muscles of the legs, easing away tension, improving the circulation of blood and lymph and freeing contracted joints. Work through the whole sequence on one leg and foot before repeating it on the other side.

1 Sitting down on the floor, with one knee bent slightly, stroke the leg with both hands from ankle to thigh in one long continuous movement. Begin the stroke as close to the ankle as you can reach. Repeat several times, moving around the leg slightly each time to stroke a different part. Try to establish a rhythm for the strokes which you can maintain throughout the whole sequence.

2 Massage the knee, stroking around the outside of the kneecap to begin with, then using circular pressure with the fingertips to work around the kneecap more firmly.

3 Knead the calf muscle with both hands, using a firm petrissage movement to loosen and release any tension in the muscle.

4 Continue kneading on the thigh, working over the top and outside areas with alternate hands. While the leg is still raised, do some soothing effleurage strokes up the back of the leg from ankle to hip.

5 Raise the leg, supporting its weight with your hands under the knee. Rotate the ankle five times in each direction.

6 Gently bring your foot over the other leg. With one hand on top of the foot and one underneath, stroke up the foot from toes to ankle. Repeat the action three times.

7 With the thumbs, apply circular pressure over the ball of the foot. Work in lines from the inside of the foot to the outer edge. Repeat three times.

8 Supporting the foot with one hand, continue the circular pressures over the raised instep, working from the inner to the outer edge. Repeat three times.

9 Still holding the foot with one hand, make a loose fist with the other and firmly rotate your fist over the instep. Work thoroughly into the arch.

10 Massage each toe individually. Slowly stretch the toe between the thumb and finger: pull gently, moving your fingers up the toe each time, until you reach the tip.

11 Repeat the effleurage strokes of the foot, with one hand over and one under the foot, working from toes to ankle several times.

MASSAGE WITH A PARTNER

Probably the best way to improve and deepen a relationship is to increase caring physical contact, and massage is an ideal approach. The ability to ease tensions and deeply relax your partner is a very satisfying form of giving. Helping someone to release tension and feel better does not have to be limited to your life partner of course; there are other members of the family, friends or colleagues who can all be helped in this way, and a better rapport will be developed with them, too.

Being massaged by someone else means that you can let go of your muscles completely. It does require trust to do so, and if you are massaging a person you do not know too well, be sensitive to this. Massage practitioners are well aware that they are being given permission to make a deep contact with their clients, and that this is a privilege that must not be taken for granted.

Make sure that you have created the right environment for a truly relaxing massage. Check that your partner is warm and comfortable and take a few moments to make contact and accustom them to your touch before you begin. Do not press harder than is comfortable for your partner and, of course, take great care never to inflict pain while you are massaging, at any time.

WHOLE BODY MASSAGE

A successful massage benefits and relaxes both body and mind, and careful preparation helps you to achieve this aim. Creating a nurturing ambience, preparing all your equipment and oils, and approaching the session in a calm and relaxed manner will give you confidence in your abilities and inspire trust in your partner.

The sequence shown on the following pages is a comprehensive, top-to-toe massage based on Swedish techniques and adapted for home practice. As a beginner you may find the full sequence too tiring at first. Until your hands and wrists build up their strength and you get used to positioning your own body comfortably to perform the massage, it is best to work on just a few parts of the body, such as the back of the legs, back and shoulders, or to perform fewer movements on each part of the body.

Your partner will find it more relaxing if you perform one or two types of movement thoroughly, rather than changing the strokes after a few seconds to cover all the steps. Always include effleurage strokes to begin and end a sequence, and never leave the body unbalanced – if you work on one leg or arm, you should repeat the same movements on the other side of the body.

Exchanging a regular basic massage is a luxury for both giver and receiver. However, you should not attempt to remedy specific problems: if in any doubt at all, seek the advice of a doctor or trained practitioner before you begin.

Pour a little oil into your palms at the beginning of the massage and oil your hands lightly again as you begin each new sequence of movements. You may need to replenish the oil more frequently if you are working on areas of very dry or hairy skin.

Establish contact with your partner by placing your hands on their body, and begin the massage with some smooth and flowing effleurage strokes.

THE FULL MASSAGE SEQUENCE

The front of the body
1 Legs
2 Feet and ankles
3 Arms and hands
4 Chest, shoulders and neck
5 Face
6 Abdomen and waist
The back of the body
7 Legs and buttocks
8 Back and shoulders

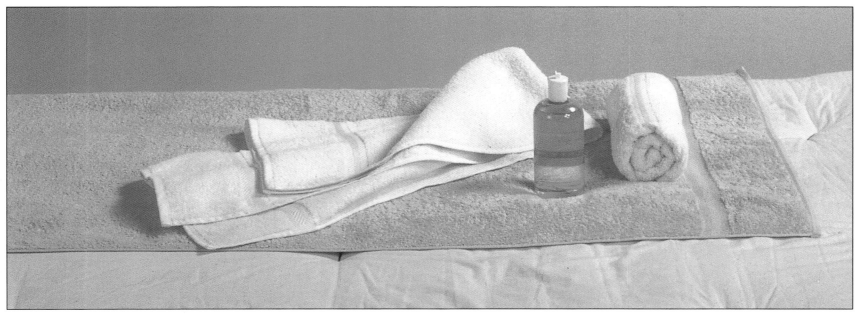

Have several towels ready, so that you can cover areas of the body not being worked on. A rolled towel behind your partner's neck or knees is often helpful.

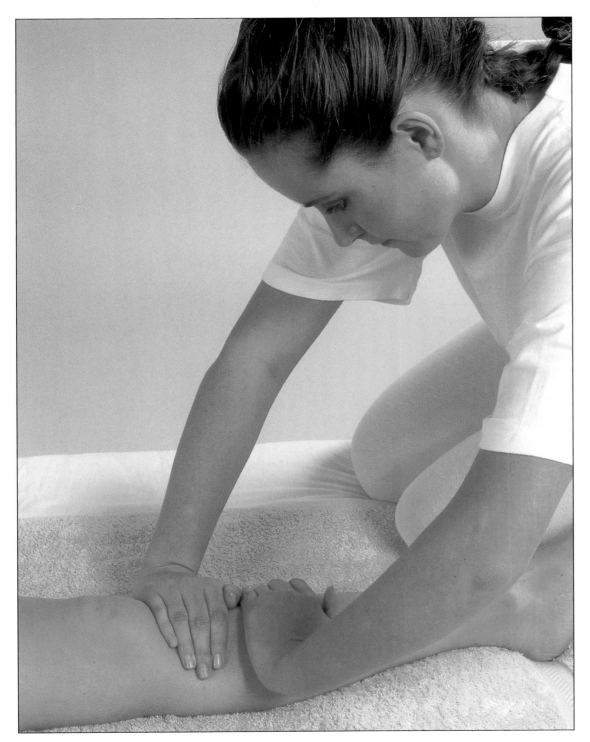

YOUR POSTURE AND BREATHING

A good posture will help you to perform fluid strokes and remain relaxed throughout the session, without straining your own body. Maintain a good, firm balance whether you are kneeling or standing, using your leg muscles to ease your body back and forth with your strokes. Keep your knees relaxed and your spine straight. Remind yourself to relax your shoulders and let your arms hang loosely so that your shoulders, elbows and wrists are flexible at all times. Keep a space between your arms and your body to avoid hunching your shoulders.

Deep and easy breathing will replenish your energy, allow tense muscles to open and relax, and bring vitality to your strokes. Synchronize your breath with your strokes to deepen the effects of your massage.

CAUTIONS: Never massage directly on top of the spine, though working down each side of the bony spinal column is fine, and produces many benefits.

There are occasions when giving a massage is not appropriate. Avoid massaging anyone suffering from any of the following conditions:

- heart condition
- high blood pressure
- bacterial or viral infection
- nausea or abdominal pain
- severe back pain which may originate in the spine, especially if there are shooting pains in any of the limbs
- temperature or fever
- open wound or skin infection
- cancer
- post-operative recovery

If you are in any doubt at all, it is always best to check with a doctor.

Pay attention to your posture as you perform the massage. By maintaining a balanced and relaxed position, you will avoid straining your own body.

THE FRONT OF THE BODY

The full massage begins with the front of the body, so your partner should lie face up with cushions or rolled towels behind the head and neck, and wherever they are needed for support.

THE LEGS

Since legs carry the full body weight, the bones and muscles in the legs are the largest and strongest we have. A good leg massage not only helps to relieve strain and tension in the legs themselves, but can benefit the well-being of the whole body. It's not unknown for backache to be traced to problems in the legs, and for a good leg massage to help alleviate the pain.

Leg massage stimulates the circulation of blood and lymph, and done regularly it helps to prevent varicose veins. Any congestion in the lower legs will be lessened with effleurage movements taken up toward the lymph nodes at the back of the knee and in the groin. If legs feel puffy or swollen to the touch, use only the gentlest of pressure.

Complete the whole sequence of movements on one leg and foot before moving around your partner to work on the other side.

CAUTION: You will need to take certain precautions if your partner has varicose veins. Never knead or put any pressure on varicose veins, and only massage the part of the leg higher than the area with the vein (that is, closer to the heart); never massage on or below the vein.

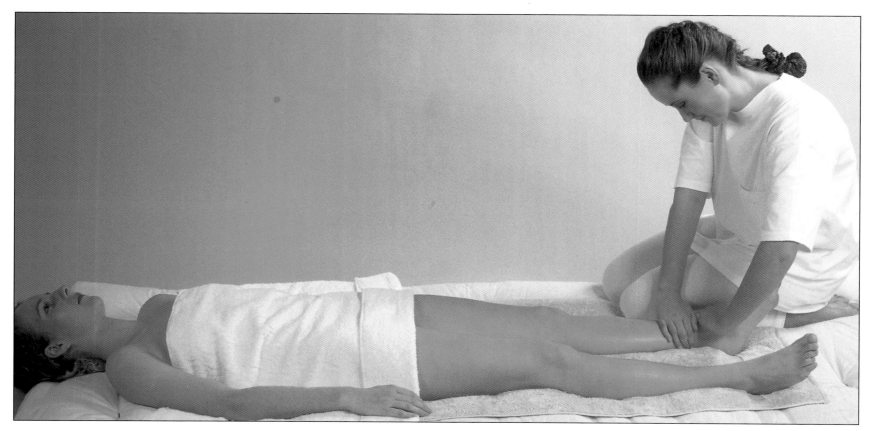

1 Kneel beside your partner's left ankle. Start with your hands crossed over the ankle, in readiness to begin several long effleurage strokes. You will need more oil if the legs are particularly hairy or dry, but don't add too much in the first instance.

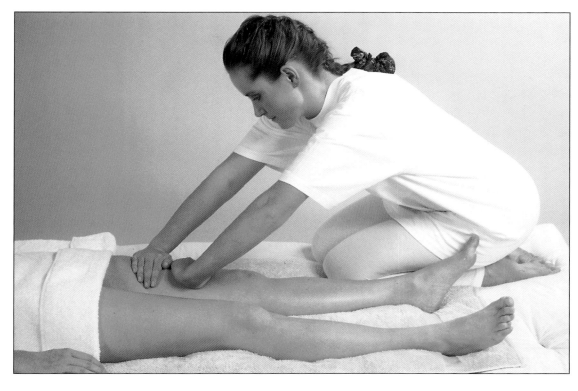

2 Keeping your hands crossed over the leg, slide the palms up the front of the leg, over the knee and up to the thigh, in one long, continuous, sweeping movement to oil the front of the leg evenly.

Rose oil is one of the most effective for promoting an overall feeling of well-being.

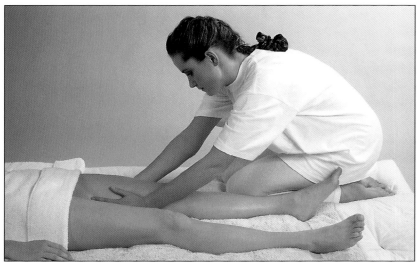

3 Turn the hands outwards around the hip, separate them and bring them back down each side of the thigh.

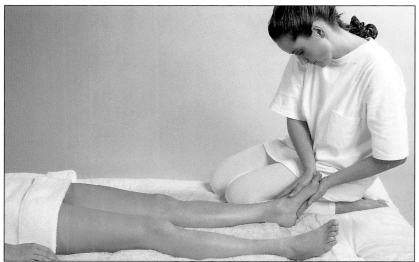

4 Continue to sweep the hands back to the ankle, and then over the foot to the toes. Then place your hands crossed over the ankle again, ready to repeat the entire movement. Use some more oil if necessary, and this time use slightly firmer pressure on the upward stroke, then lighter again for the return. The stroke is smooth and continuous throughout. Repeat the sequence over the whole leg once again.

THE THIGHS

Firm massage on the larger muscles around the thighs can dispel tiredness and stimulate a sluggish lymphatic system, which brings many health and vitality benefits.

1 Bring both hands up to just above the knee and move them up together, pressing the muscles firmly towards the upper thigh. You should be applying enough pressure to see movement in the muscles.

2 At the top of the thigh, separate the hands and, using lighter pressure, come down either side of the leg to the knee.

3 Begin kneading the inner thigh with both hands. Squeeze, then release the muscles, picking up and rolling them as you do so. Continue the kneading action over the top and outer thigh.

4 Now use a hacking movement all over the thigh area. Briskly strike the area with the outside edge of your hands, one hand after the other, using short, sharp, quick movements.

5 Continue with cupping all over the thigh, working quickly. Expect quite a loud cupping sound, but remember to check with your partner that the strokes are not too powerful.

6 Beginning at the knee, do some effleurage strokes up to the top of the thigh, sweeping the hands outwards and back down to the knee, to soothe the area after the series of stimulating movements.

THE KNEES

Move smoothly down the thigh to the knee, where you need to work very gently over the bony area.

1 Place both hands just below the knee. Lightly massage around the kneecap, using your fingertips to work gently into the muscles around the bone. Maintain the massage for about 2 minutes.

3 Support the back of the knee with your hands and use your thumbs to circle gently around the kneecap, working downwards. Return to the top of the knee and repeat three times.

THE CALVES

When you have finished working on the knee, do some more effleurage strokes, sweeping them up from the ankle to just below the kneecap and back down to the ankle, and repeating them several times.

2 Starting with your thumbs above the kneecap, and with your hands under the knee for support, slowly draw them around the outside of the kneecap and release. Repeat this movement three times.

1 Knead the calf muscles. Squeeze and release them, working from the ankle up to the knee.

2 Lightly and quickly pinch the fleshy part of the calf with the fingers and thumbs, one hand after the other. Check with your partner that you are not pinching too hard; although it does need to be felt to be effective, this should not actually be painful.

4 Raise the height of your hands above the knee. Work around the kneecap with one hand, loosening the muscles with your thumb and fingers. Use gentle circular rotations to cover the area thoroughly. You may find it easier to support your wrist with the other hand, to prevent your wrist from becoming tired.

3 Using the outside edge of both hands, alternately and rhythmically strike the calf muscles, working up and down the entire length of the lower leg, but keeping away from the back of the knee and the bony shin area. Keep the hacking action short and brisk.

4 Starting at the ankle and crossing your thumbs on top of the shin for support, make semicircular kneading movements with loose knuckles, working up and down the calf. Finish with some relaxing effleurage movements from ankle to thigh.

THE FEET AND ANKLES

A foot massage is particularly relaxing after the legs have been worked on. It can alleviate anxiety and stress, stimulate the circulation and nervous system, promote sleep and energize anyone feeling tired and lethargic. There are thousands of nerve endings in the foot, especially on the sole. Try to include the ankles too, to improve their flexibility.

Change the pressure of the strokes to suit your partner, remembering that deeper pressure tends to revitalize, whereas gentle strokes increase relaxation. When working on the feet it is best to use only a very little oil, otherwise your hands will slide around and tickle. If your partner's feet are hot and sticky, use a little talcum powder instead.

Before starting, you may wish to raise the knee slightly with a rolled towel, to relax the muscles around the knee and in the lower back.

1 Kneel at your partner's feet. Starting with your hands at the ankle, gently slide them towards the tips of the toes and then release them. Repeat several times. If you are using oil, apply it with this stroke.

2 With the heels of your hands, give a good stretch to the top of the foot. Draw the hands towards the sides of the foot to give the stretch. Repeat a few times, working slightly further down the foot.

3 Supporting the foot in both hands, find the furrow between each tendon and, using small circular movements, work both thumbs up the tendons towards the ankle. Repeat three times on each tendon.

4 Resting the thumbs across the top of the ankle, work the fingers right around the ankle bone, using light, circular movements.

5 Lightly tap the toes with your fingers to build up some gentle friction.

6 Knead the foot firmly, working particularly well into the arch. You will need to use different parts of the hand, such as the heel, knuckle and thumbs.

7 Supporting the lower leg with your left hand, gently rotate the ankle three times in each direction, without forcing it.

8 Give the foot a gentle stretch backwards and forwards, to relax and flex the tendons. Supporting the back of the lower leg, use your other hand at the toes to push the foot gently away from you. To reverse the stretch, take the hand over the top of the foot and press the foot down, still supporting the lower leg with the other hand.

9 Finish the foot and ankle sequence with some long sweeping effleurage strokes from the top of the foot up the lower leg and back down to the foot, to help reintegrate the foot and the leg. Repeat several times, varying the pressure.

The oil extracted from the geranium plant has stimulating and uplifting properties.

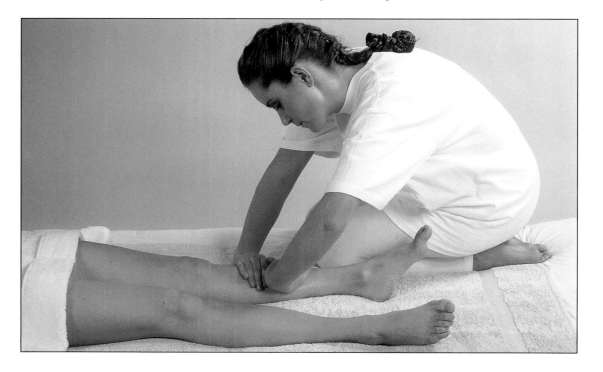

THE ARMS

Arms and hands can hide the most powerful emotions. Tight, clenched arms and hands often reflect insecurity, self-protection and unresolved anger. Whether the posture is intentional or subconscious, tension in the arms can cause headaches, neck pain and aching shoulders. Don't be put off if your partner's arms are slim and bony; there are still important muscle areas there.

Mellow and peaceful lavender oil has been valued for centuries for its calming qualities.

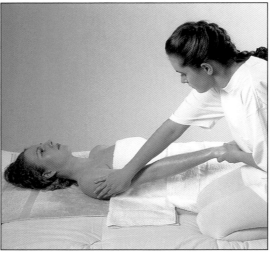

1 Kneel halfway along your partner's right side. Holding the wrist with your left hand, lightly oil the arm using effleurage strokes, starting from the wrist and sweeping your hand up around the shoulder and down again. Repeat three times.

2 Changing hands, so that your partner's wrist is supported in your right hand, use the left hand to stroke gently from the wrist to the shoulder, and back down again. Repeat several times.

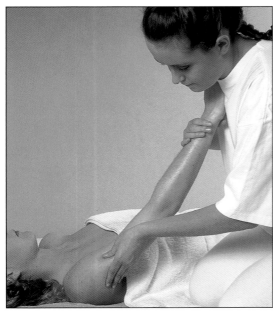

3 Lift the arm and rest the hand on your right shoulder ready to start kneading. Support your partner's wrist with your right hand and use your left hand to knead the muscles of the upper arm lightly.

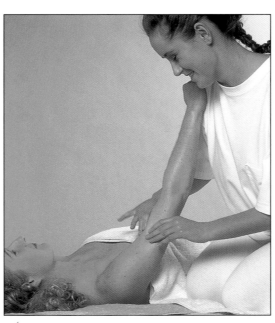

4 Keeping your partner's hand supported by your shoulder, use the fingers of both hands to continue the kneading.

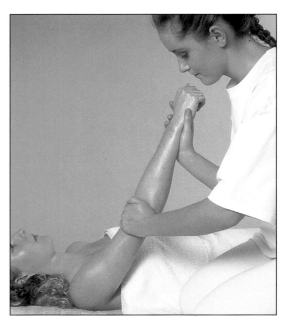

5 Still holding the arm across the front of your chest with your right hand, do some effleurage strokes from the elbow up to the shoulder and back down again. Repeat three times.

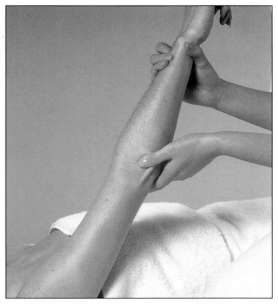

6 Bend your partner's arm and rest the right hand on the left shoulder. Using the outside edges of your hands, do some short, brisk hacking on the outer and under sides of the arm.

7 With your partner's arm still bent, firmly knead the muscles of the upper arm with your right hand, using the left hand to keep your partner's arm stable.

8 Holding the wrist for support with your right hand, work around the outside of the elbow with your fingers and thumb, using smooth circular movements and covering the area thoroughly. As the elbows can get very dry, you may need some more oil.

9 To encourage further relaxation, hold the wrist with your left hand and do some effleurage strokes up and down the top of the forearm. Keep the pressure fairly firm.

10 Repeat these effleurage strokes on the inside of the forearm.

11 Rest your partner's elbow back on the towel. Supporting the weight of the lower arm in your left hand, use your right hand to knead the inside of the forearm, starting from the wrist. When you reach the elbow, glide gently back to the wrist to begin again. Repeat three times. Finish the arm with a few effleurage strokes.

THE HANDS AND WRISTS

A hand massage is surprisingly effective, and is almost on a par with having the feet massaged. Our hands are in almost constant use throughout the day, at work, for household chores or in leisure activities, acting simultaneously as multi-purpose tools and shock barriers. Not surprisingly then, a lot of tension creeps into the hands, and a massage is a reminder of how good it feels to relax them completely. Massaging the arms and hands increases suppleness and dexterity, and can liberate and relax not only the muscles but also the pent-up emotions, as your partner starts to feel the wonderful sensation of letting go.

1 Support your partner's hand in both hands and gently use the thumbs to knead the palm. This should be a continuous, circular action, with the thumbs alternately applying the pressure.

2 Rest your hands under your partner's wrist and use the thumbs to stroke outwards around the wrist. Then work with the thumbs up the inner forearm toward the elbow, using circular movements.

3 Turn your partner's hand over, supporting the wrist with one hand. Massage over the back of the wrist with your thumbs, taking care to keep the movements light as you work over the bone.

4 Stroke up in between the tendons on the back of the hand with your thumbs, from knuckles to wrist, using light, small circles. Repeat twice between each tendon.

5 Sweep your hands alternately up from the wrist towards the elbow, applying a fairly firm pressure with the inside edge of the hands. Repeat several times.

6 Come back down to the hand and gently stretch the back of the hand, drawing your own hands out towards the sides.

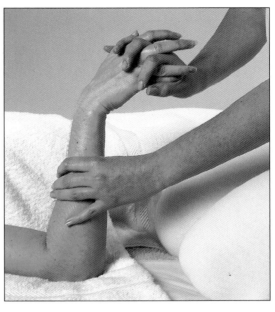

7 With one hand, make circular pressure movements around the finger joints, starting at the tip. When you have worked around all joints, rotate each finger twice. Stretch each finger to release the joints.

8 Raising your partner's lower arm and supporting it with your left hand, clasp your partner's hand with your right hand and gently rotate it in a half-circle, three times in each direction.

9 Still supporting the lower arm, thread your fingers between your partner's and gently bend the wrist backwards and forwards three times, making sure that the wrist joint is not forced.

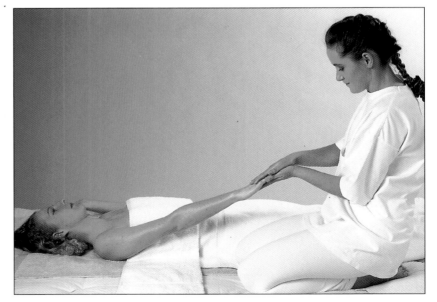

10 Finish the arm and hand sequence by stroking the entire length of the arm and hand with some soothing effleurage from palm to shoulder.

11 Hold your partner's hand between both of your palms for several seconds, then release, lowering the arm gently. Move around to kneel on the other side and repeat the arm and hand massage on the left.

THE CHEST

It's not only the hours spent sitting hunched over a desk that tighten and contract the chest muscles – emotional tension is often stored in the chest area, and clutching a car steering wheel, carrying heavy shopping and poor posture all have a cumulative effect.

Before you begin, check whether your partner's neck would be more comfortable with a small cushion or folded towel under the head. Kneel behind your partner's head to start the sequence.

1 With the flat of the hands placed on the chest, fingers pointing away from you, place your left hand on top of the right. You will be doing reinforced effleurage on the right side of the chest first.

2 Sweep your hands over the chest, towards and around the right shoulder, keeping the left hand over the right, in a continuous effleurage stroke. You should apply enough pressure to press the chest and shoulder towards the floor, so that they release as you end the stroke. Repeat three times.

3 Continue the effleurage stroke, sweeping both hands around and up the right side of the neck. Repeat the sequence twice more, starting from the centre of the chest each time, as in step 1.

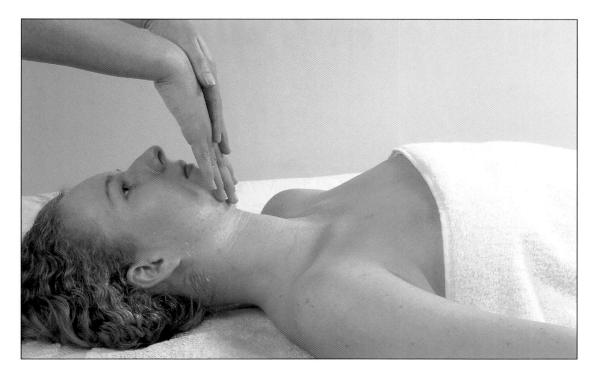

4 Repeat once again, but this time finish by bringing both hands up to the jawline with the fingers resting lightly under the centre of the jaw.

Use rosemary oil to help strengthen the mind in times of mental fatigue and emotional stress.

5 With both hands, knead the fleshy area in front of the armpit. Pick up and release the muscles, squeezing them from one hand to the other.

6 On the same fleshy area, lightly pinch the surface muscles between the thumb and first finger. Alternate the hands swiftly in a rhythmical action, checking with your partner that this causes no discomfort. Repeat steps 2 and 3 to soothe the area you have worked on, then repeat the whole sequence on the left side of the chest.

THE SHOULDERS AND NECK

Tension in the chest can exacerbate inflexibility and stiffness in the neck and shoulders. We tend to raise the shoulders towards the ears, until they become set rigid with tension.

The uplifting properties of rose oil can help ease strain in the neck caused by nervous tension.

1 Place both hands fairly firmly, side by side, over the front of the chest.

2 Sweep them out towards each shoulder with firm effleurage strokes, taking them over the shoulders, around under the upper back and up the back of the neck.

3 When you take the movement around the back and the neck, gently lift the weight of your partner to give the muscles a gentle stretch.

4 With your fingertips, work with circular pressures up the back of the neck to the base of the skull. These should be small, firm rotations, which you can feel easing taut muscles. You should spend some time on this area, which is often extremely tense; take the trouble to release as much tension as possible.

5 With loose fists, use the knuckle area to ripple your fingers in semicircular frictions all over the upper chest. Keep the half circles fairly small and apply firm pressure on the fleshier area, but avoid working directly on the collarbone.

6 Bring your loose fists under the upper back and continue to knead behind the shoulders and around the base of the neck.

7 Finish with several effleurage strokes, starting at the front of the chest and stroking the hands over each shoulder and up behind the neck.

THE FACE

The face constantly mirrors our health and emotions. Stress and tension are reflected in a furrowed brow, and lines around the eyes, mouth and jawline. A facial massage can soothe away headaches, anxiety and exhaustion and replace them with a feeling of serenity. It improves the circulation, giving the skin a healthy glow.

If your partner wears contact lenses, make sure they are removed before you start a face massage. Use a little light oil, and don't let it get too near or go in the eyes, mouth or nose. Make sure the hair is held securely away from the face and neck in a soft hairband. Keep the hands relaxed. You may be surprised to find that the face is less fragile than it looks and you can apply quite deep pressure without causing discomfort.

1 Kneel at the top of your partner's head. With your hands placed over the collarbone, pointing away from you, begin with some gentle effleurage strokes.

2 Sweep your hands out across the shoulders, keeping the pressure light.

3 In a continuous movement, bring your hands up around the back of the neck to the nape; pause for a moment, increasing the pressure slightly with the fingertips, then release and lift your hands away. Repeat this effleurage sequence at least three times.

4 Bring your right arm across the front of your partner so that the hand supports the left shoulder. Using light upward strokes, sweep your left hand up from the top of the shoulder, up the side of the neck to the edge of the jaw. Repeat three times.

5 Now repeat this movement on the other side of the neck.

6 Starting with both hands over the front of the chest, fingers pointing toward each other, lightly sweep the flat of one hand up the front of the neck to the jaw, flicking the hand away when you get there. As you flick the first hand away, bring the second up, so that you stroke with alternate hands. Repeat this stroking and flicking movement several times.

7 Bring both hands up to the front of the jaw. Alternately sweep one hand and then the other up along the jawline towards the ear. Repeat the movement several times.

8 Briskly tap the length of the jawline using the middle and ring fingers, starting from the centre front and working towards the ears. This should have a stimulating effect, so keep the patting movement quick and fairly firm.

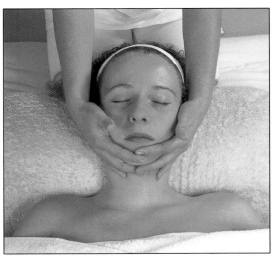

9 Afterwards, soothe the area by cradling the face gently with both hands. Pause for several moments, then release the hands.

10 Bring your hands up to the forehead. Loosely interlock your fingers, and using the palms, apply gentle pressure over the forehead. Slowly unlock the fingers to release. Repeat three times.

11 Starting with the third finger of each hand placed on the bridge of the nose, stroke out over the brows towards the temples at each side of the forehead. Come up the forehead a little and, starting again with both fingers at the centre front, repeat the strokes out towards the hairline. Repeat a couple of times more, bringing the fingers higher up the forehead each time, until the whole forehead is covered.

12 To finish, place your hands on each side of your partner's head, and pause for a few seconds before lifting them away.

THE ABDOMEN

Many people feel exposed and vulnerable when baring their abdomen, so you will need to be particularly sensitive to your partner when it comes to this part of the massage. Start with very gentle strokes, but try to be confident, as a gentle touch which is also tentative can feel unnerving for your partner.

Massage of the abdomen calms the nerves and can soothe stomach aches if they are caused by tension, poor digestion or period pains. It also stimulates the digestive organs so that elimination is improved. You should wait for at least an hour after your partner's meal before giving an abdominal massage.

Rhythm

It helps to start and finish the massage by focusing on your partner's breathing, so that your strokes coincide with their body's natural rhythm. To begin, try slowly stroking your hands up from the lower abdomen to the chest on inhalation, and down the sides of the body on exhalation.

1 Kneel beside your partner at hip level. Make contact by gently placing your hands together in a diamond shape over the lower abdomen, pointing towards the head. Keep the fingers together and the hands relaxed. Ask your partner to breathe into the abdomen so you can feel it expand and contract. Work with the breath.

2 Slowly slide your hands up the centre of the abdomen until you reach the ribs, making sure the pressure is even and not too firm.

3 Continue the movement by sweeping the hands out and around the sides of the waist. As you take them out from the ribs towards the sides, you can apply a little more pressure, so that you feel the muscles being drawn outward.

4 Return to the starting position, with both hands placed on the lower abdomen, and repeat this continuous movement several times.

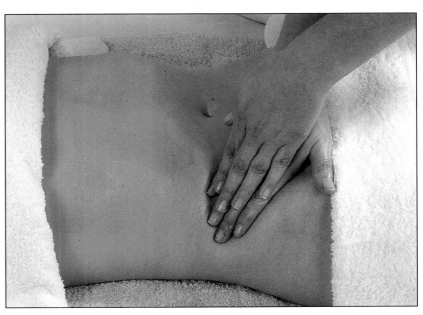

5 Place both hands on the right-hand side of your partner's lower abdomen, ready to circle the navel. Rest your left hand over the right for support.

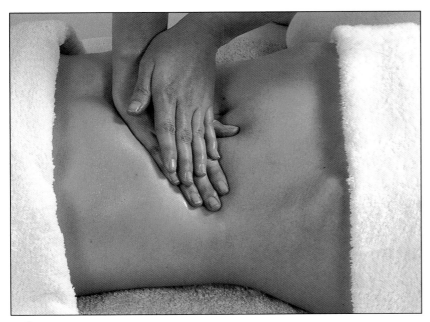

6 Stroke upward, keeping the left hand over the right, until you reach the ribs. The pressure can be quite firm to stimulate the digestive system. Keep the stroke smooth and continuous.

7 Continue the stroke by bringing your hands across under the ribs, and down the left side of your partner's abdomen. Repeat the navel-circling movement three times, each time returning to the centre of the lower abdomen, and always working up the right side, across and down the left side.

MASSAGE WITH A PARTNER

THE WAIST

Your movements around the waist area should be firm and stimulating, but lighten your touch as your hands cross the abdomen to reach the opposite side of the body.

1 To begin the massage, knead around the waist area by squeezing and releasing the flesh from one hand to the other.

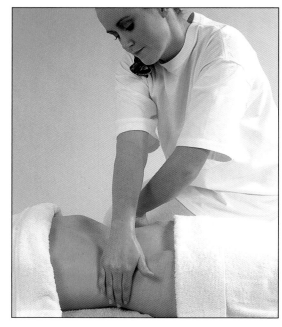

2 Cross your hands over your partner's waist so the palms are grasping each side of the midriff. Briskly draw them up the sides of the waist, uncrossing them as they meet and turning the palms to travel down the other side. Draw up again and recross the hands to reach your starting position. Repeat four times.

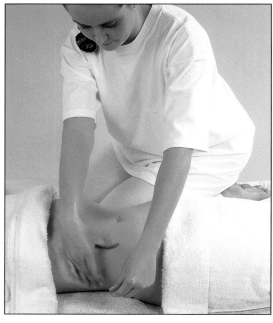

3 Starting at the far side of the waist, lightly pinch the flesh between fingers and thumbs with brisk, short movements. Repeat the same movement on the other side of the waist.

4 Lightly cup the side of the waist, keeping the pace fast and stimulating, but at the same time checking that it is not causing discomfort. The action should not be painful, but should be enough to increase the flow of blood to the area.

5 Working on the top of the hip area, squeeze and release the flesh in a kneading movement, using deep and stimulating pressure.

6 Finish the massage of the abdomen by repeating the soothing effleurage strokes from the beginning of the previous sequence. End with both hands placed over the centre of the abdomen, fingers pointing towards the head. Hold for a few seconds before lifting your hands off.

THE BACK OF THE BODY

Ask your partner to turn over on to their front, ready for you to start work on the back of the legs and buttocks.

THE LEGS

Effleurage on the legs can stimulate other body functions and can help improve their efficiency. Poor circulation and a sluggish lymphatic system can be considerably improved by a good leg massage. Tiredness and heaviness in the legs is alleviated and your partner should be left with a feeling of renewed energy.

Complete the whole back of leg massage on one leg before moving around to the other side of your partner to repeat the sequence. Cover the leg you have worked on with a towel to keep the muscles warm.

1 Start by kneeling at one side of your partner's ankles. You should be able to work on both legs from the same side quite easily. Begin by working on the leg furthest away from you and cross your hands over the back of the ankle.

2 Stroke up the leg in a smooth and continuous movement, with the right hand leading the left. When you reach the back of the knee, pause for two or three seconds.

3 Carry the stroke up the leg and cross the hands at the top of the thigh, keeping the pressure even and light throughout the movement.

4 Bring your hands back down the sides of the leg to the ankle. Repeat the sequence three times, each time increasing the pressure slightly.

CAUTION: You will need to take certain precautions if your partner has varicose veins. Never knead or put any pressure on varicose veins, and only massage the part of the leg higher than the area with the vein (that is, only massage closer to the heart); never massage on or below the vein.

THE UPPER LEGS AND BUTTOCKS

The backs of the legs and buttocks offer plenty of scope for massage techniques. Most people can take plenty of firm massage on the larger muscles in the thighs and buttocks. The fleshy parts are ideal for kneading and squeezing, and firm pressure can feel wonderfully satisfying. Kneel at your partner's side and work on the leg opposite.

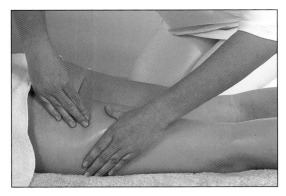

1 Using a firm kneading movement, squeeze and release the back of the thigh muscles, working up to the buttock. You should be able to pick up quite a large area of muscle between the hands.

2 With the outside edge of the hands, do some short, sharp hacking movements. Alternate the hands in a quick, repetitive action. Continue the hacking all over the back of the upper leg and the buttock.

3 Continue working on the upper leg and buttock, with some cupping. The cupping action should be short and fast to stimulate the whole area.

4 With loose fists, briskly pound the top and outside of the thigh. You can use the backs of your fingers or the outside edge of the fists. Use a firmer knuckling action over the buttock area.

5 Follow this sequence of friction movements with soothing effleurage strokes from the back of the knee to the top of the thigh, sweeping out and back down the leg to the knee.

THE CALVES

Move down to kneel beside your partner's ankles, and work on the calf of the same leg, lightly oiling your hands again if necessary.

1 Start with both hands on the back of your partner's ankle. Smooth your right hand up towards the knee, keeping your left hand on the ankle for support. Keep the pressure light on the back of the knee.

2 As you continue the stroke, taking your right hand up towards the top of the thigh, slide your left hand up the lower leg to the back of the knee. Try to do this in one single, flowing movement.

3 Without pausing, bring your right hand in one stroke back down the leg. Slide the left hand off the knee, so the right hand can continue down to the ankle. Repeat the effleurage stroke at least three times.

4 Knead the calf with both hands, working from the ankle up to the knee, but do not knead the back of the knee. If the muscles are tight, this action may feel uncomfortable, so do ask if the pressure is right.

5 Do some short, sharp pinching movements all over the calf muscle, again checking that you are not hurting your partner.

6 Supporting your partner's leg in the left hand, slide your right hand up from the back of the ankle to the knee. Keep the pressure as firm as is comfortable. Repeat three times before gently lowering the leg.

7 With your thumbs together, start at the back of the ankle and work up the back of the calf to the knee, applying pressure firm enough to release tightness in these muscles. When you reach the back of the knee, lighten the pressure and sweep your hands back down the sides of the leg to the ankle. Repeat three times, then repeat the effleurage strokes from the beginning of the whole sequence to soothe the leg.

Orange essential oil is known to act as an antidote to water retention in the lower legs.

THE BACK AND SHOULDERS

The back is an area of great strength and mobility, and it is the main supportive structure of the body. It therefore warrants more attention than most other areas. By working on the back, you can reach nerves affecting every part of the body.

Full back massage, with emphasis on the spine and lower back, greatly alleviates the effects of stress throughout the body, enhancing physical and psychological well-being. Smooth, flowing strokes stretch the muscles and tissues around the contours of the back, and help to restore flexibility for health and mobility, while stronger strokes along the spinal muscles and over the lower back bring deeper relief to aching or knotted muscles.

With your initial effleurage strokes, concentrate on finding areas of tension and tightness.

1 Before you begin to work on the back, make sure your partner is comfortable, lying face down with arms resting beside the face. Support the forehead with a rolled towel, and if it is helpful use a pillow or rolled towel under the chest. It is a good idea to have the hair clear of the back of the neck, secured in a soft band. Kneel beside your partner's hip.

2 Starting at the lower back, begin the effleurage strokes. With thumbs crossed to connect the hands together, move slowly up the centre of the back, putting firm pressure on the fingertips.

3 Take the stroke up to the top of the back in a continuous movement.

4 Without a pause, separate the hands at the top of the back, sweeping them out and around the shoulders.

5 Continue the stroke, bringing both hands down the sides to the lower back, ready to begin again. Repeat this effleurage sequence three times, oiling your hands each time.

THE SHOULDERS

Work through this sequence from your original position, then move to the other side of your partner and repeat the steps on the other shoulder.

1 Using your thumbs on each side of the spine, start level with the shoulder blades and make circling pressure movements. Work quite firmly into the muscles, but remember to ask your partner if the movement is causing them any discomfort.

2 Continue working up each side of the spine until you reach the nape of the neck. Keep the amount of pressure even, and try to maintain a steady rhythm for the stroke.

3 Carefully bring your partner's right arm across the hollow of the back and clasp the hand with your left hand. The shoulder blade should now stick out slightly. With your right thumb, make circular pressure movements over the shoulder area. Strong muscles support the shoulder blade and you can work firmly under the bone to release tightness here.

4 Having replaced your partner's arm, work in small circular movements from the base of the neck out over the shoulder. Rest your left hand over your right to increase the pressure.

5 Continue the movement around to the shoulder blade, using firm pressure to release tension in the muscle. Repeat steps 1–5 on the other side of your partner's body.

THE BACK

Avoid using percussion strokes such as hacking and cupping on the kidneys, which are level with the waistline in the centre of the back.

1 Knead the far side of the back firmly with both hands, beginning at the outer side of the waist. Pick up, roll and release the muscles, alternately pressing one hand towards the other. Continue kneading up the back until you reach the shoulders. Start again at the waist but this time come closer to the spine and repeat the line of kneading up the back. Repeat on the near side of the back – you should be able to do this without altering your position.

2 Using the outer edges of your hands, briskly and rhythmically hack from the lower back up to the shoulders, but avoid the bony shoulder blade. Try to visualize each side of the back divided into three sections so that you cover the whole back thoroughly.

3 Start cupping from the lower back, working upward and across the shoulders. The action should be quick, with alternate hands striking the back briskly.

4 Repeat the effleurage strokes from the beginning of the back massage sequence to soothe the back. Repeat several times.

THE SPINE

It is important to remember never to massage directly on the spine itself, although working down each side of the spine can be highly beneficial.

Lemon oil can refresh and clarify thought. Use it on the back for a thoroughly uplifting massage.

1 With loose fists, and thumbs crossed for support, push the top of the hands up each side of the spine to the nape of the neck.

2 Uncurl the fingers when you reach the nape and sweep them back down the sides of the back. Repeat these strokes three times.

3 Starting at the lower back, place the thumbs on either side of the spine, resting your hands at either side of the back. Rotate the thumbs in small circles, travelling up the sides of the spine until you reach the hairline. Use firm pressure. Reverse the movement, circling your thumbs back down each side of the spine.

4 Starting at the lower back, use loose knuckles, crossing your thumbs over each other for support, to work up either side of the spine and back down again. Repeat twice.

5 Using the backs of your hands and starting at the lower back, push up either side of the spine to just above the waistline. Then sweep your hands outward and back down around the hips. Repeat three times.

6 To finish the massage, repeat the effleurage strokes from the beginning of the sequence, starting at the lower back and working up the back, around the shoulders and down again to the lower back, in a continuous sweeping movement.

A full back massage using oil of neroli will soothe anxiety and encourage a sense of peace.

ᴵNSTANT MASSAGE

Do you come home at the end of the day with your neck and shoulders feeling as if they were set in concrete? Does stress leave your back stiff and aching? Anyone who experiences the physical tensions that accompany stressful situations will find that massage is one of the most successful ways to relax painful, knotted muscles. Most of us almost unconsciously rub tense, aching spots to obtain some instant relief; correctly performed, massage can have a wonderful effect on tense muscles and on our whole sense of well-being, even if you only have a few minutes.

One of the great advantages of massage is that it can be adapted to virtually any situation. You can relax most completely if you have a partner to massage you, but it is almost as effective if you do it on yourself. Some of the strokes are versatile enough to apply not only at home but also in the workplace or even on a bus, since it is not essential for you to be naked or even partially clothed for your tired, aching muscles to be massaged. Massage through clothes can be very effective, though a little more pressure may need to be applied. You can apply a particular sequence of strokes to ease specific muscular aches or, if you have a little more time, combine several of the sequences that follow for a relaxing but quick and easy massage, any time, anywhere.

10-MINUTE MASSAGE

Sometimes the idea of having the tension in your shoulders and neck instantly massaged away is particularly tempting. Without stopping to find the right place and time to undress, a shoulder massage can be done with the minimum of disruption. There are times when the best therapy you can give your partner is a quick shoulder and back massage while sitting comfortably on an upright chair. It can be done through light clothing if that is simpler, and there is no need to use oil if you prefer not to.

1 Ask your partner to sit astride a chair, facing the back. You can offer a folded towel or cushion for comfort. Standing behind your partner, begin by leaning on your forearms so that your weight presses down gently on to the fleshy part of the shoulders.

2 With your partner leaning forward, use effleurage strokes from the bottom of the shoulder blades, up the back and out over the tops of the shoulders, to finish at the tops of the arms. Repeat four times.

3 With a firm petrissage, use both hands to knead out along the shoulders from the sides of the neck to the upper arms.

4 Starting as far down the lower back as you can, work up the spine with small circular friction strokes. Continue up the sides of the neck to the base of the skull, then glide back down and work up again, this time moving out over the shoulders as you reach the top of the back.

5 Move around to the side and tilt your partner's head forward, supporting it with one hand. With the thumb and finger of the other hand, grasp the neck firmly and massage with circular movements, working up the neck and into the base of the skull.

6 Working from behind your partner again, massage the back of the head with both hands, coming over the forehead and down to the temples with small circular pressures, moving the scalp against the skull. Lighten your touch at the temples.

7 First on one side, and then on the other, do some hacking across the fleshy parts of the shoulders and upper back, using the outer side of your hands to make short, brisk movements. Keep your wrists and hands very relaxed.

8 Continue with a brisk cupping action across each shoulder, working on one side at a time. Remember to keep your wrists and hands relaxed as you work.

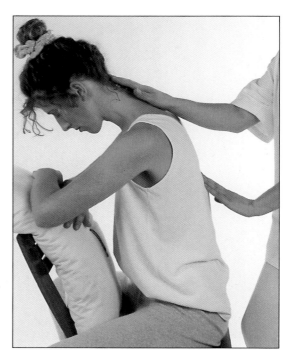

9 Finish the sequence by gently stroking down the entire back with one hand following the other. Repeat five times, with each stroke lighter than the last.

INSTANT SELF-MASSAGE

Self-massage is a quick and effective way to relieve tension or pick yourself up at any time of day, whether you need to relieve a particular group of tired, aching muscles, or to re-energize yourself when you have run out of steam.

SIMPLE REVITALIZER

At any time during a busy day your energy can flag. If you need to be bright and alert for a meeting, a long drive, picking up the kids or going to a party, give yourself an instant "waker-upper" with this short routine.

The balancing effect of lavender oil makes it a wonderful stress-beater.

1 Use a fast kneading action on the arms, working rapidly from the wrist to the shoulder and back again with a firm squeezing movement, to invigorate the arm and shoulder.

2 Rub swiftly up the outside of the arm to stimulate the circulation. Repeat several times, working in an upwards direction each time, to encourage blood flow back to the heart. Repeat the sequence on the other arm and shoulder.

3 With the fingers and thumb of one hand, firmly squeeze the neck muscles using a circular motion.

4 With the outside edges of the hands, lightly hack along the front of the thighs, using a rapid motion. The hands should spring up from the muscles.

5 Rub the calves vigorously to loosen the muscles and to get the blood moving. If possible, do this with the legs bent. Make each stroke from the ankle to the knee, using alternate hands. Finally, stand up and shake your whole body, to let go of any remaining stiffness and tension.

HEAD REVITALIZER

Headaches can have a multitude of causes, such as spending too much time in front of a VDU, anxiety, insomnia, fatigue or sinus congestion. However, the most common cause is tension arising from periods of stress. Use this self-massage sequence to help ease a headache, whatever its cause. You can also use it at any time to increase your vitality and help you to focus your mind.

Nutmeg essential oil has a warming, stimulating effect, and can help relieve nervous fatigue.

1 Use small, circling movements with the fingers, working steadily from the forehead down around the temples and over the cheeks.

2 Use firm pressure and circle the fingertips slowly to ease tension out of all the facial muscles.

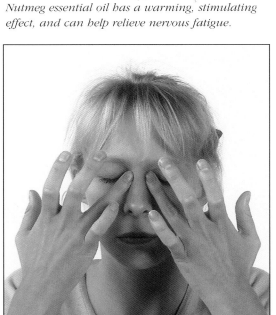

3 Press gently around the eye socket, by the nose, using the third finger of each hand.

4 Smooth firmly around the arc of your eye socket beneath your brow bone.

5 Work across the cheeks and along each side of the nose, then move out to the jawline where a lot of tension is held. Try not to pull downwards on the skin – let the circling movements help to smooth the stress away and gently lift the face as you work.

TENSE NECK EASER

As you get tired, your posture tends to droop, making your neck and shoulders ache. Practise these movements and help release any mounting tension in these areas before your shoulders become permanently hunched up.

Ginger oil will help counteract all manner of aches and pains.

1 A simple movement is to shrug your shoulders, exaggerating their contraction by lifting them up as far as possible and then letting them drop down and relax completely.

2 Firmly grip your opposite shoulder with your hand and use a squeezing motion to loosen the tension in the muscles. If your working arm starts to ache, rest for a moment before continuing.

3 Move slowly along the shoulder, squeezing the flesh firmly several times between your fingers and the ball of your hand. Repeat on the opposite side, using the other hand.

4 With the fingers and thumbs of both hands, grip the back of the neck and squeeze in a circular motion to help relax the muscles leading up either side of the neck. Work up to the base of the skull and down again to the shoulders.

5 To work more deeply into the neck, move the thumbs in a circular movement across the neck and right up into the base of the skull. You will feel the bone as you apply moderate pressure.

TONIC FOR ACHING LEGS

Any occupation that involves long periods of standing still can create real problems for circulation in the legs, leading to tired, aching limbs, swollen ankles or cramp. It is, of course, essential to try to move around as much as possible, but a quick self-massage at the end of the day can help considerably in reducing stiffness and sluggish blood flow in the legs. Remember to take extreme care if your partner suffers from varicose veins. Do not apply pressure to the vein itself, and massage only on the part of the leg above the vein (that is, nearer to the heart); never work below the vein.

1 Start a leg massage by working on the thighs, so that any fluid retention in the calves will have somewhere to go as the upper leg relaxes. Knead the flesh of the thigh between the fingers and thumb, squeezing with each hand alternately and working from the knee to the hip and back. Repeat on the other thigh.

2 Around the knees, use a similar kneading action, but for a lighter effect use just the fingers and work in smaller circles.

3 Bend your leg, and if possible raise the foot on a chair or handy ledge. With your thumbs, work on the back of each calf with a circular, kneading action. Repeat a few times, each time working from the ankle up the leg to the knee.

4 Squeeze the foot, loosening up the muscles and gently stretching the arch. Use firm pressure with your thumb to stretch the foot. Repeat on the other foot.

CHEST AND ABDOMEN RELEASER

The front of your body is an area where emotional tension is often stored; bottling up your feelings can create tight muscles across your chest or in your abdomen. Massage treatments on these areas often trigger the release of deep-seated emotions, and need a skilled, sensitive approach. Self-massage is, however, very helpful, both in easing tense muscles and in helping to recognize where stored tensions lie. An awareness of the effects of stress is the first step towards letting go of it.

1 Using the thumb and fingers, take a good grip of the pectoral muscles leading from the chest to the shoulder, and knead them firmly.

2 Be careful if you have any tenderness in the lymph glands under the armpits. Women should also go gently if they have tender, swollen breasts; for example when pre-menstrual.

3 Using a couple of fingers, feel in between the ribs for the intercostal muscles, and work firmly along between each rib, moving the fingers in tiny circles, repeating on each side.

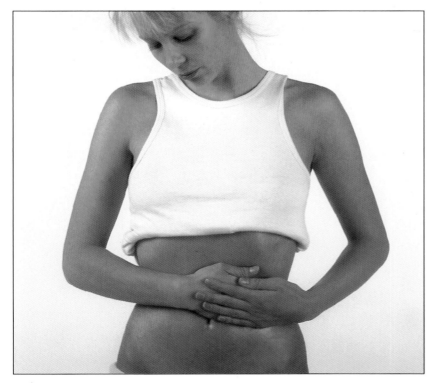

4 Place your hands on your abdomen, and, pressing gently, work around slowly in a clockwise direction.

5 If it is comfortable, repeat twice with increasing pressure; ease off if this becomes painful. Working in this direction encourages digestive and bowel action.

OFFICE MASSAGE

Massage is a highly versatile skill, and can be applied in many situations. When one of your work colleagues complains of tense, aching shoulders or back, you can do something about it to alleviate the pain.

A FIVE-MINUTE MASSAGE

No special equipment is needed for this simple yet effective massage sequence. It can be done at a desk, and can be wonderfully effective in refreshing and re-energizing people. You can work on people when they are fully clothed and still seated at their desk.

2 Knead both shoulders at the same time, with a firm squeezing movement; adjust the pressure you use according to the amount of clothing and the degree of discomfort your partner is experiencing.

1 Standing behind your seated colleague, place your hands on both their shoulders, with your thumbs towards you and fingers to the front.

3 Using your fingers, knead in small circles up and down the back of the neck. Always try to support the head with your free hand while you are working on the neck.

4 Place your forearms over the shoulders and press down with your body weight to squeeze and stretch the trapezius muscles.

5 Move the forearms outwards to the shoulders, maintaining a firm pressure all the time.

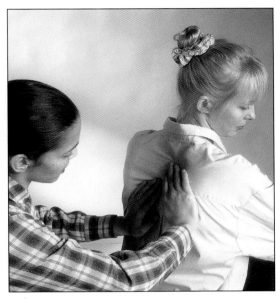

6 Using your fingers, make firm circling motions down the back, to either side of the spine.

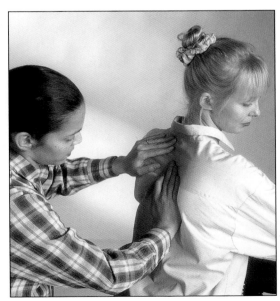

7 Allow the fingers to sink into the muscles around the shoulder blade. Repeat on the other side.

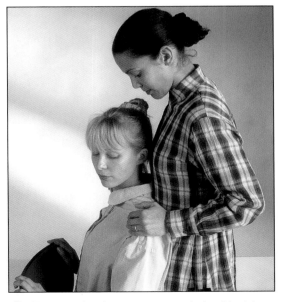

8 Place your hands on your partner's shoulder joints and press back towards yourself. This movement will give a gentle stretch to the upper chest.

9 With care and balance, you can do this stretch with your leg pressing into your colleague's back.

NECK AND SHOULDER RELEASER

The build-up of tension and pain in the neck and shoulders are common symptoms of today's pressured and stressful work environments. This is a common cause of headaches at work. A tension headache is often experienced as a "tight band" around the head. It is thought that such head pains are caused by a change in blood pressure, which occurs when the muscles tense and restrict the normal flow of blood to the head and face. The pain is usually accompanied by muscular tension around the upper part of the body. The following quick-and-easy routine is designed for the workplace and will provide relief to the accumulating tension in the neck and shoulders.

1 Have your partner sit on a chair with proper back support to encourage a straight spine. This will allow for better energy flow. Make contact with your partner's shoulders and take a minute to tune in and see how your partner feels. Be aware of any tension in the shoulders and listen to the breathing.

2 Grip and hold the trapezius muscles (the muscles of the shoulders and neck) on either side of the neck. Squeeze these muscles a few times, combining your thumbs and fingers in a rhythmic "kneading" action. There may be tension initially but this will slowly dissolve. Work within your partner's pain threshold.

3 To encourage your partner to relax into the treatment, take a firm grip of their upper arms; ask your partner to breathe in as you lift the shoulders up and breathe out as you allow the shoulders to drop back down again. Repeat three times.

4 Keep your own shoulders, wrists and hands relaxed and "soft". Use a gentle hacking action with the sides of your hands and move rhythmically across the shoulders and base of the neck. Increase the intensity and power of the hacking as the muscles relax and your partner's discomfort, if any, disappears.

CHEST AND NECK RELEASER

Sitting hunched over a desk all day can lead to shallow breathing and a stiff neck. This is caused by the contraction of chest muscles, which in turn can also exacerbate inflexibility and stiffness in the neck and shoulders. We tend to raise the shoulders towards our ears, until they become set rigid with tension. This 5-step routine will open up the chest, encouraging better breathing and posture, and relax the muscles in the neck, which can also relieve stress-induced headaches. Before starting this sequence, ensure your partner is sitting comfortably, with both feet on the ground so that the spine is aligned.

1 Stand behind your partner and take hold of the lower arms.

2 Ask your partner to take a deep breath in; on the exhalation bring the elbows towards each other behind the back. Repeat three times. This will open up the chest and encourage better breathing.

3 Stand at your partner's side. Ask your partner to relax and drop their head forward into your left hand. Hold the forehead until you feel your partner has given up control of the neck. Using the fingers and thumb of your right hand, gently squeeze the muscles of the neck, patiently working from top to bottom.

4 Keep your left hand on your partner's forehead and with your right hand support the neck into a forward stretch, opening up the back of the neck and the spine.

5 Place your right arm across your partner's shoulders. Apply a gentle lifting movement with your forearm as your left hand guides the head back on to your forearm. This stretches the front of the neck.
Caution: The base of the skull and neck must always be supported by your forearm to prevent too strong a movement backwards, which could cause injury.

$\mathscr{H}$EALING MASSAGE

Massage can evoke many beneficial changes within the body, mind and spirit of the whole person. As well as relaxing stiff and aching muscles, it is a powerful treatment precisely because it works on both physical and psychological levels, and because it is able both to relax and invigorate the person receiving it. As the vicious circle of tension between mind and body is broken down by massage, the specific symptoms to which the tension gives rise can be alleviated.

To touch, caress and hold is a natural response to emotional or physical pain, and it is a practice found in every culture. During a massage, soft, flowing strokes calm and soothe the nervous system, stimulate the nerve-endings in the skin, and warm and loosen the superficial tissues. Deeper strokes remove tension from muscles and increase suppleness and mobility. Blood and lymph circulation is boosted, so that vital nutrients reach all the cells and toxins are eliminated. Revitalizing strokes invigorate energy levels and leave the skin with a healthy glow. Breathing deepens as the person becomes more relaxed and energized, increasing the intake of oxygen into the body and the expulsion of carbon dioxide from the lungs. Calm, still holds will enable the person to relax deeply and discharge pent-up feelings of stress.

HEADACHE AND TENSION RELIEVER

One of the most common symptoms people experience when they are under stress is a tension headache; for some, this can become almost a daily pattern and may lead to migraine attacks. Any treatment should be given at the earliest stage, and massage is no exception. Just a few minutes of these soothing strokes may prevent major muscle spasm and pain.

1 Ask your partner to lie down and kneel or sit just behind them, with their head in your lap or on a cushion.

2 Using your fingertips, work with alternating circular friction strokes on the muscles on either side of your partner's neck.

3 Continue circling, this time with both hands working at the same time, around the side of the head and behind the ears.

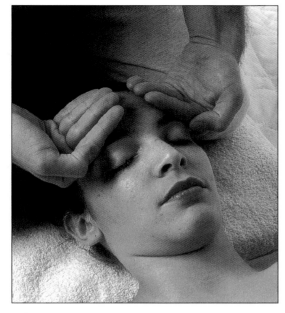

4 Smooth tension away from the temples with the backs or sides of your hands, using some gentle effleurage strokes.

5 Gently draw the hands outwards across the forehead to soothe away worry lines.

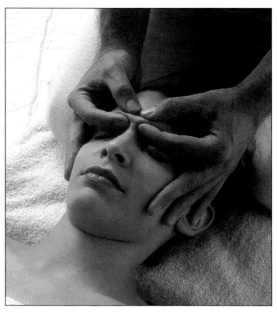

6 Pinch and squeeze along the line of the eyebrows, picking up the flesh between finger and thumb. Reduce the pressure as you work outward.

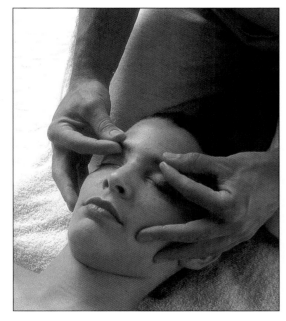

7 These muscles may be quite tender, so check with your partner and do not apply more pressure than is comfortable.

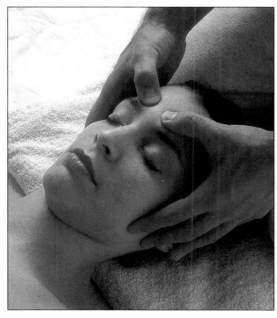

8 With your thumbs, use steady but firm pressure on the forehead, working outwards from between the eyebrows.

9 Work across the brow to the hairline using your thumbs. This covers many acupressure points and will release blocked energy.

SLEEP-ENHANCING FACIAL SOOTHER

If your partner has frequent problems with sleeping, or simply carries a lot of tension around in the facial muscles, this soothing programme may help. Apart from acting as an aid to relaxation, working on these muscles will smooth out worry lines and re-invigorate the face.

1 Kneeling behind your partner's head, with their head resting comfortably on a cushion, place both your hands under the neck. Pull very gently on the neck muscles, creating a little traction to stretch out the neck and head.

2 With your fingertips, make small circling friction movements along the jawline and over the cheeks. Use firm pressure but, as with all massage, avoid causing any discomfort. Try to work symmetrically, using both hands at the same time.

3 Pull gently with the fingertips and stretch the ears, working around from the earlobes to the top of the ears and back again.

4 Apply circling friction movements with your fingers or thumbs on the temples and forehead, lightening your touch as you work up the temples.

5 With the palms of your hands, smooth across the forehead, soothing the area you have worked on and easing out tension and worry lines.

6 Continue this movement, but now working your hands towards you, and extend it by stroking up into the hair to complete the sequence.

POOR CIRCULATION

Poor circulation to the extremities is quite common in cooler climates, and particularly in elderly people or those who do very little exercise. It can lead to more serious conditions, such as phlebitis or thrombosis, so it should not be neglected. Cold hands and feet can be warmed up initially by rubbing them briskly between your hands: the friction both warms the skin and stimulates the blood supply.

1 Using a little oil, massage the palm of the hand with a steady circular movement of the thumb.

2 Squeeze down each of the fingers to stretch and loosen the joints, pushing towards the palm. Repeat steps 1 and 2 several times.

3 To stretch the foot, place both hands with the thumbs on top and fingers underneath, keeping a firm grip.

4 Move the thumbs outward, as if breaking a piece of bread. Repeat the movement several times, keeping the fingers still while moving your thumbs.

FLUID RETENTION

Excess fluid in the tissues, or oedema, can have a variety of causes. Fluid retention in the thighs and hips in women is often associated with a build-up of toxins, as is cellulite. In hot weather most people find that fluid retention is aggravated. A general detoxifying programme of diet, exercise and massage will usually help.

Massage the legs and thighs to improve the local circulation and so bring more blood and oxygen to the muscles. Firm effleurage movements are particularly helpful, always done in a direction towards the heart.

Inadequate circulation to the muscles is also a cause of cramp, especially if it comes on with exercise or effort. It is probably most common in the calves, but the acute and painful contraction can occur in any large muscles. For frequent leg cramps, regular massage of the legs and thighs is recommended. Essential oils such as juniper, lavender, marjoram, rosemary or black pepper will help to dilate the local blood vessels and encourage increased blood flow. Night cramps are likely as a combination of reduced circulation, tiredness and stress, and the whole person needs to be treated to alleviate this painful symptom.

1 To improve circulation in the legs, place your hands on your partner's thigh and stroke upwards to the buttock several times using smooth effleurage movements. Keep the pressure light but steady, letting one hand follow the other.

2 Move your hands down to the calf and stroke up to the back of the knee a few times. Repeat these two steps, always starting the massage on the upper leg and always stroking towards the heart.

MASSAGE AND EXERCISE

Professional sportspeople value massage very highly. Used before exercise it helps to prepare the body for an increase in activity, not only by warming and loosening the muscles and joints – thereby helping to prevent cramp and injury – but also by stimulating the system physically and mentally. After an exercise session, massage speeds up the elimination of waste products, particularly lactic acid, by stimulating the lymphatic system. The accumulation of these toxins during exercise is the cause of much of the stiffness and pain that may otherwise be experienced afterwards.

STRAINS AND SPRAINS

A burning sensation under the skin is likely to indicate that muscles, fibres or ligaments have been strained – stretched beyond their natural limits. This is often the result of exercising without an adequate warm-up, or of over-exertion. A pre-exercise massage and warm-up routine will help prevent strains. Gently massaging the affected area will help speed recovery.

Sprains are more serious and are caused by violent wrenching of a joint, most commonly the ankle, wrist or knee. The surrounding muscles, ligaments and tendons may also be damaged and the affected area may be extremely painful and swollen. Apply an ice-pack or cold compress for 15–20 minutes to reduce the swelling. After this you can start to massage the area gently, taking care not to work directly on the swelling. Rest the joint as much as possible and use a support bandage.

A serious sprain should always be checked by a doctor in case a bone has been fractured, and a sprained knee always requires medical attention.

1 Avoid working directly on the swollen area (in this case the ankle). Start with gentle effleurage strokes working from the knee towards the thigh. Massaging in the direction of the lymph nodes in the groin will help drain away the fluids that have accumulated around the injured joint. Lightly stroke back to the knee. Repeat several times.

2 Help your partner to bend the affected leg. Continue the effleurage strokes on the lower leg, this time working from the ankle to the knee, alternating your hands. Repeat several times, then gently squeeze the calf with one hand, while the other supports the foot.

3 Concentrating on the ankle area, stroke extremely gently all around the ankle with short upward movements. Check that this is not causing discomfort.

ALLEVIATING BACKACHE

Back strain is the most common source of debilitating pain. Most sports put strain of some kind on the legs, buttocks and back, and previous injuries can make the back prone to recurrent pain. Falls and awkward landings are an inevitable part of many sports, but you should take care to avoid inappropriate or excessive exercise wherever possible. You should never subject your back to unnecessary strain. A regular and thorough back massage, particularly before exercise, can greatly reduce the likelihood of injury by loosening up the muscles and improving suppleness. Always consult a doctor, osteopath or chiropractor if you are in any doubt about the seriousness of a back problem.

ESSENTIAL OILS AND BLENDS FOR SPORT

Before exercise
For supple, toned muscles:
black pepper; ginger; rosemary; lavender; cypress; juniper; peppermint; grapefruit; orange.

To aid the respiratory system for aerobics:
eucalyptus; peppermint and rosemary; geranium.

For mental preparation before an event:
rosemary; lemon; lavender and chamomile.

To improve circulation:
rose and palmarosa.

After exercise
To soothe and prevent aching muscles:
eucalyptus; ginger and peppermint.

To eliminate stress following a competition:
lemon; nutmeg; clary sage; orange.

ALLEVIATING CRAMP

It is usually underused or ill-prepared muscles that go into cramp during exercise. Frequent cramps may indicate poor circulation or a deficiency of calcium or salt. Massage will improve circulation and alleviate the pain.

1 To relieve calf cramp, have your partner lie face down with the foot of the affected leg supported on your leg or a small pillow. Gradually apply direct thumb pressure into the centre of the cramped calf muscle for 8–10 seconds.

2 Do some effleurage strokes, working from ankle to thigh and back down again.

3 For hamstring cramp, raise the ankle on a small pillow and begin by massaging up the back of the thigh using alternate hands in slow, rhythmical stroking movements. Then apply static pressure to the middle of the thigh with the thumbs, holding for 8–10 seconds.

4 Firmly knead the calf muscle. Squeeze, press and release the muscle using one hand after the other. Finally, do some soothing effleurage strokes up from ankle to thigh and back down again.

SELF-HELP CRAMP STRETCHES

Cramp is a sudden and involuntary contraction of a muscle, and you can help to alleviate the pain by stretching the muscle gently to help it relax.

1 A good way of dealing with calf cramp is to sit down with the affected leg straight and stretch the toes towards you. Hold this position for 8 seconds, then release. Repeat a few times, until the spasm seems to be lessening, then knead your calf muscle using firm pressure. When the muscle feels relaxed, switch to effleurage strokes, working up the leg.

2 For hamstring cramp, lie down flat on the floor, with the affected leg raised and the other knee bent. Stretch the muscle by pulling the thigh gently towards the chest. Firmly stroke up the back of your thigh for 8–10 seconds. Start to knead the back of the thigh until you feel the muscles begin to relax. Finally, stroke over the area to soothe it.

TENNIS ELBOW

Pain on the outside of the elbow may be due to inflammation of the tendon resulting from overuse. It may be caused by sporting activities, but can also result from digging in the garden or lifting heavy objects. Avoid repeating the activity for a week or two to allow the inflammation to subside.

1 Support your partner's wrist in one hand and use soothing effleurage strokes along both sides of the arm, stroking from the wrist to the elbow and back again. Repeat several times.

2 Rest your partner's hand against your side. Continue to work up their arm, from the wrist to the elbow and back, making small circular movements with both thumbs, paying particular attention to the muscles in the forearm.

3 Secure your partner's hand in yours, and with your other hand supporting their elbow, flex your partner's elbow forward.

4 Bring the hand back, to give the tendons that are attached to the bones a good stretch.

SENSUAL MASSAGE

As well as releasing stresses and tensions from the muscles, massage is a wonderful way to enhance a relationship by increasing caring, sharing touch. If your relationship seems to have got into a rut and sexual energy is low, you can revitalize yourselves with some soothing massage strokes.

The skin is so highly sensitive that it is able to transmit and receive loving messages and feelings conveyed through the hands, nourishing not only the body but the mind and emotions. Massage can become a means of deep communication, a way to show how much you care for each other.

It is important to take a little extra time to create the right environment so as to make the whole experience a real treat – time for you both in a hurried world. Make the room extra warm and wear minimal clothing or undress fully, covering your partner with warm towels if necessary. You may want to play some of your favourite soothing music. Arrange soft lighting or, better still, work by candlelight.

Gentle effleurage strokes should be the mainstay of a sensual massage. Use a little more oil than usual to help the strokes flow more easily.

Intuition will play a large part in your massage, as you discover which areas have the strongest impact on your partner's senses. It isn't just the most obvious erogenous zones that bring pleasure: pay attention to the back of the neck, scalp, solar plexus, the inside of the elbows, and the hands and feet, to make the massage a highly pleasurable and sensual experience for both of you.

1 Using gentle effleurage strokes, place your hands on either side of the spine and glide right down the back from the shoulders. Move your hands out to the side and up the back again. Repeat several times, making your hands soft and pliable so that they mould and encompass the shapes and curves of your partner's body.

2 Kneeling beside your partner's hips, stroke down the centre of the back with one hand following the other smoothly, as if you were stroking a cat.

3 As one hand lifts off at the lower back, start again with the other hand at the neck in soothing, languid strokes.

4 Place both of your hands on your partner's upper back and stroke outwards in a fan shape. Shape your hands to the sides of the body, then draw them down before sliding them lightly around and back to the centre of the back.

5 Work down the back, including the buttocks, repeating the fanning action.

▶

6 Use a firm, steady circling action on the buttocks. These are large, powerful muscles that may be able to take quite firm pressure if your partner desires it, but avoid giving any discomfort.

7 Stroke up the back of the legs, with one hand after the other, in a smooth, flowing motion.

8 As one hand reaches the buttocks, start on the calf with the other hand, keeping a steady rhythm. This overlapping stroke creates the sensation of many hands caressing the body, and feels particularly wonderful on the legs and arms.

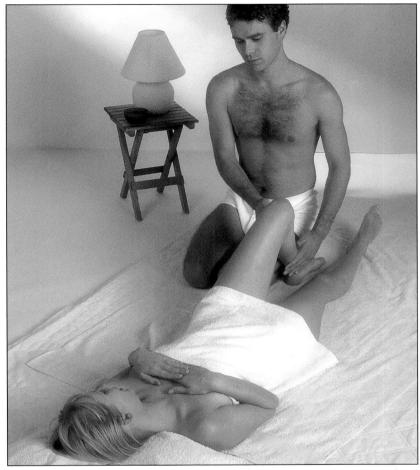

9 Turn your partner over and stroke up the front of the legs; bend the knee to help the muscles relax completely.

10 Continue the movement up the leg, using both hands to stroke from the knees up to the thighs.

11 Effleurage may also be used on the front of the body, kneeling behind your partner's head. Be careful not to press in with your thumbs. All these movements should make for a truly sensual experience, and help put your partner back in touch with their body – and maybe yours too.

SENSUAL OILS

When choosing essential oils for sensual massage, the most important consideration is personal taste. The massage will not be a pleasurable experience if either of you finds the blend of aromas disagreeable. Allow an intuitive choice to guide you in making a blend of aromas that you both find appealing.

There are, however, a few oils that seem to have a universal appeal: jasmine, rose, rosewood, sandalwood and ylang ylang. These oils are the embodiment of luxury and are indeed some of the most precious. They have a warming and enveloping quality, freeing the mind and opening it to the exotic and romantic. To add spice and stimulation to your chosen blend, add either black pepper or frankincense.

ENHANCING YOUR MASSAGE

Once you have achieved a good grounding in the basic techniques of massage, you can further enhance your skills by using a massage couch, and by experimenting with the use of additional pillows.

WORKING AT A COUCH

While some people prefer to kneel and give a massage at floor level, working at a couch increases your mobility, as you can move more freely when on your feet. This puts less stress on your posture, enabling you to bring length to your spine and neck and a relaxed width to your shoulders. As with the kneeling position, your movement should come from the lower half of your body to avoid strain on your back.

There are many different types of massage couch to choose from, designed for various styles of massage and in a wide price range. It is important to choose a couch built to the correct height for you: if you stand with your fists loosely clenched and let your arms hang down by your sides, you should be able to rest your knuckles comfortably on the surface of the couch. The width of a massage couch should be a minimum of 65–80cm/26–32in, in order to support the whole body securely and allow sufficient space for the arms to relax on the couch. The length is normally a minimum of 180cm/72in. Foam padding, covered with vinyl, should be firm but comfortable.

A face cradle can be added to the table, or a face hole cut into its surface, to enable the head and neck to be supported straight. Some people find it difficult to lie in a prone position as it necessitates an awkward angle of the neck.

If you are planning to set up a mobile massage practice and want a portable, folding couch, it is important to choose one that is easy to carry. You will need to find the right balance between stability, strength and ease of transportation.

USING PILLOWS AND TOWELS TO EASE TENSION

Postural tension remains in the body even when your partner is lying down on the couch to receive a massage. A prolonged period of resting on a flat surface can even exacerbate physical strain, especially in the major joints of the body. The more you massage, the more you will be able to see where someone is holding tension. For example, an individual may have a particularly swayed lower back, indicating stress in the pelvic region, or the neck may be contracted or sore, making it extremely difficult to lie comfortably. Using pillows or rolled towels to support key areas of the body can ease the structural tension, enabling your partner to relax and enjoy the highly beneficial experience of massage to the full.

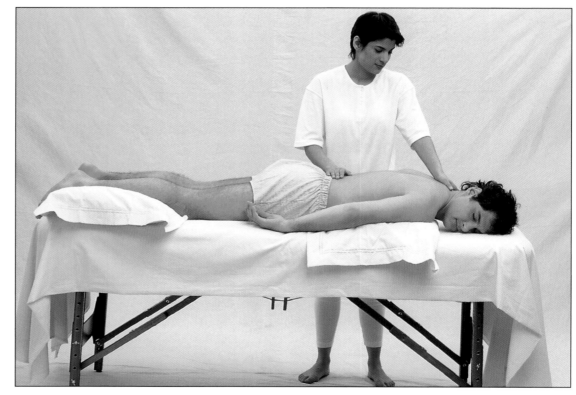

1 When your partner is lying in a prone position, place one pillow just below the knees. The benefit of taking the strain out of these joints will further relax the pelvis and lower back. A pillow under the front of the chest will allow the shoulders to fall forwards, opening up the upper back and creating space between the shoulder blades. The added support will also help to lengthen and relax the back.

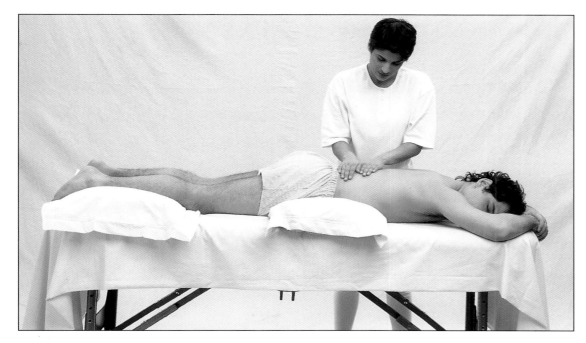

2 Pain in the lower back may be caused by an excessive curve in the base of the spine, or a chronic pattern of tension in the pelvic region. A pillow placed supportively under the abdomen can redress the postural imbalance during the massage, helping the lumbar region to relax under your touch.

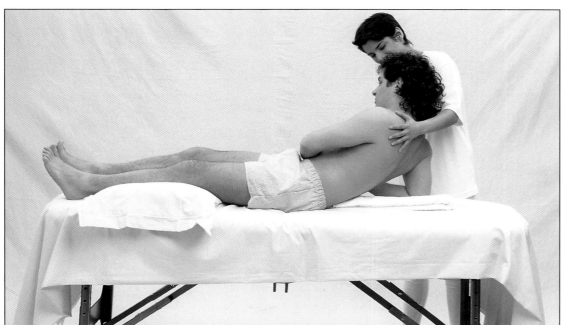

3 Tension in the chest and ribcage can cause muscles to contract, pulling the shoulders forwards so that they are unable to rest on the table during massage. Ease this uncomfortable posture by placing a towel, folded into a thin strip, under and along the length of the spine. This will enable the chest to expand and the shoulders to fall back. Help your partner into the supine position so that the towel remains in the correct place.

4 Constriction in the muscle attachments at the base of the skull will shorten the neck muscles, causing the head to contract backwards. Bring a sense of length and relief to this area by placing a thin, folded towel under the ridge of the skull to lift the head slightly upwards and to extend the neck.

BODY ENERGY AND AURIC MASSAGE

Knowledge of the body's auric and energy vibrations has always existed in spiritual and healing practices, but has been largely ignored by modern medicine and science. The influence of this subtle energy field on our health and well-being can be explored through massage, which can bring to the aura the benefits of healing and balance, helping to protect the physical body from ill-health and emotional disturbance.

1 Make sure your partner is lying down comfortably and feeling warm and safe. Take time to become still and meditative within yourself by focusing your attention on your own body and breathing. This will help your hands tune into subtle energy vibrations. Begin with a session of healing holds to bring a sense of unity to the body and restore equilibrium to the mind.

2 Raise your hands to shoulder level and let them drift down with sensitivity, to feel the edge of the aura as a tangible but subtle vibration. Enter this energy field, resting your hands, without weight, on your partner's body. Tune into your partner's essential energy, and hold until intuition tells you to move your hands.

3 This polarity hold brings a sense of integration and balance to both sides of the body. When at your partner's left side, place your left hand on the right shoulder and your right hand on the left hip. Imagine a current of energy passing between your hands.

4 Healing holds on the legs and feet can help to earth the physical body and stabilize the emotions. Start with a hip and foot hold to connect the whole leg. Then place your right hand over the knee, keeping your left hand on the hip. Finally, place your left hand over the knee while cupping your right hand beneath the sole of the foot.

5 When your partner is calm, massage the aura in smooth, slow, rhythmic strokes towards the feet, working down the body and over the limbs one at a time. Do this three times: start by clearing the spiritual plane (45–60cm/18–24in above the body), then move to the emotional plane (15–20cm/6–8in) and finally, to the physical level (5–7.5cm/2–3in). To finish, let your hands hover over your partner's abdomen and heart, before settling gently on the body.

USEFUL ADDRESSES

ORGANIZATIONS

Association of Physical and Natural Therapists
93 Parkhurst Road
Horley, Surrey
UK RH6 8EX
Tel: 01293 775467

Institute for Complementary Medicine
Unit 4, Tavern Quay
London
UK SE16 1QZ
Tel: 0171 237 5165

New York Institute of Massage
PO Box 645
Buffalo
NY 14231
USA
Tel: 800 884 NYIM

PRACTITIONERS AND COURSES

Champneys
Chesham Road
Wiggington
Tring
Hertfordshire
UK HP23 6HY
Tel: 01442 863351

Grayshott Hall
Headley Road
Grayshott
Nr Hindhead
Surrey
UK GU26 6JJ
Tel: 01428 604331

Henlow Grange
Henlow
Bedfordshire
UK SG16 6BD
Tel: 01462 811111

London College of Massage
5 Newman Passage
London
UK W1P 3PF
Tel: 0171 323 3574

London School of Sports Massage
88 Cambridge Street
London
UK SW1V 4QG
Tel: 0171 233 5962

Massage Training Institute
24 Highbury Grove
London
UK N5 2EA
Tel: 0171 226 5313

American Massage Therapy Association
820 Davies Street
Evanston
IL 60201
USA

Boulder School of Massage Therapy
PO Box 4573
Boulder
CO 80306
USA

The Connecticut Center for Massage Therapy
75 Kitts Lane
Newington
CT 06111
USA

Australian Natural Therapists Association
PO Box 522
Sutherland
NSW 2232
Australia

South African Institute of Health and
Beauty Therapists
PO Box 56318
Pinegowrie
22123
Johannesburg
South Africa

FURTHER READING

Nigel Dawes and Fiona Harrold, *Massage Cures*, Thorsons, 1990

George Downing, *The Massage Book*, Wildwood House, 1973

Fiona Harrold, *The Massage Manual*, Headline, 1992

Nitya Lacroix, *Massage for Total Relaxation*, Dorling Kindersley, 1991

—*Sensual Massage*, Dorling Kindersley, 1989

Lucinda Lidell, *The Massage Book*, Ebury Press, 1984

Clare Maxwell-Hudson, *The Complete Book of Massage*, Dorling Kindersley, 1988

Sara Thomas, *Massage for Common Ailments*, Sidgwick & Jackson, 1989

Jacqueline Young, *Self Massage*, Thorsons, 1992

INDEX

A

abdomen 120, 144–5, 146, 164–5
  pain relieving 82–3, 107
  pregnancy 89
abscesses 33
acne 20, 21, 22, 24, 25, 26, 27, 28, 30, 31, 32, 33, 35, 36, 56, 106
allergies 22, 27, 31
almond oil 36, 52, 53, 58, 60, 88
alopecia 106
anger 22, 23, 27, 30, 31, 33
ankles 88, 122, 132–3, 178–9
Anthemis nobilis 22, 106
anxiety 20, 24, 26, 28, 29, 30, 33, 35, 50, 82, 107
  massage 76–7
aphrodisiacs 21, 28, 43, 46, 107
appetite 20, 21, 25, 29, 30, 94, 106
apricot kernel oil 58, 88, 104
arms 95, 134–5, 160, 181
  circulation 84
  self-massage 118
arthritis 20, 21, 22, 23, 26, 27, 28, 29, 35, 49, 51, 92
asthma 19, 48, 105
athlete's foot 33, 35
auric massage 188
avocado oil 36, 58, 104

B

babies 33, 90–1
baby oil 104
back 89, 150–5, 179, 186–7
  10-minute massage 158–9
  office massage 166–7, 168
  self-massage 120
  sensual massage 182–5
barber's rash 32
basil oil 19, 35, 46, 50, 58, 76, 89, 105
bathrooms, oils for 46

baths 19, 49, 50–1, 61, 76, 78, 88, 92, 97
  after-bath treatments 52–3
bay oil 19, 35, 89, 105
bed-wetting 20, 22
bedrooms, oils for 46
benefits, physiological, of massage 102–3
benzoin oil 20, 35, 41, 42, 84, 88, 92
bereavement 23, 28
bergamot oil 14, 19, 20, 24, 35, 38, 40, 42, 44, 46, 50, 51, 54, 80, 82, 94, 97, 105, 106, 107
birth, after 89
  post-natal depression 24, 89
black pepper oil 21, 35, 40, 41, 43, 80, 82, 84, 86, 88, 92, 94, 97, 106, 177, 179, 185
blending essential oils 34, 36, 38, 43, 60, 105,
  see also dilution rates
blends, essential oils 40–3, 44
  see also individual topics
blisters 33
blood pressure 22, 32, 33, 35, 48, 50, 106, 107
body massage, whole 126–7
  see also specific parts
body oils 44, 52–3, 88, 89
boils 20, 22, 27, 32
borage oil 36
Boswellia thurifera 24
breasts 88, 165
breath, bad 20, 31
bereavement see grief
breathing
  accelerated 33
  for massage 127
bronchitis 20, 21, 23, 24, 27, 28, 29, 30, 31, 32, 33, 35, 80
bruises 24, 25, 27, 28
burns 22, 24, 27, 36
buttocks 121, 148, 184
  cellulite reduction 87
buying essential oils 17, 104

C

Caesar, Gaius Julius 100
calves 103, 131, 149, 181
  self-massage 122, 160, 163

camphor oil 17
Cananga odorata 33, 107
cancer 22
candida 30, 33
  see also thrush
candles 47, 97
carrier oils 36, 50, 104
carrot oil 36
catarrh 21, 24, 25, 26, 27, 32, 33, 80
categories of oils 39
cautions
  chest and neck releaser 169
  deep massage 112
  essential oils 19, 105
  percussion movements 113
  pregnancy 89
  spinal massage 127
  varicose veins 128, 147
  see also major references to named essential oils
cedarwood oil 10, 21, 35, 39, 42, 43, 44, 46, 47, 50, 54, 58, 80, 84, 92, 97, 105, 106
Cedrus atlantica 21, 106
cellulite 23, 24, 25, 26, 27, 35, 50, 69, 106, 121, 177
  self-massage 86–7
chamomile oil 14, 22, 35, 39, 40, 41, 50, 51, 54, 56, 58, 60, 74, 78, 82, 88, 89, 90, 92, 106, 179
chemicals in essential oils 15
chest 138–139, 141
  office massage 169
  self-massage 164–5
chicken pox 20, 33
children 39, 47
  baby massage 90–1
  oils for 28
chillblains 20, 21, 22, 24, 27, 28
chills 20, 21, 25, 29, 30, 35
cinnamon oil 35, 46
circling 110
circulation 49, 72, 86, 92, 94, 106, 107
  benefits of massage 102, 103
  massage 84–5, 95, 176, 177
  oils for 20, 21, 23, 24, 25, 27, 28, 29, 31, 32
Citrus aurantium 29, 30, 107
  C. bergamia 20, 106

C. limonum 27, 107
C. paradisi 25
C. reticulata 28
citrus oils 16, 106
clary sage oil 19, 22, 35, 39, 40, 41, 42, 43, 46, 74, 76, 78, 82, 89, 94, 97, 105, 179
cleansers, skin 55
cold sores 20, 27, 33, 56
colds 20, 21, 23, 24, 25, 26, 27, 28, 29, 30, 31, 33, 35, 48, 50, 56, 72, 74, 80–1, 106, 107
colic 20, 21, 22, 25, 28, 30, 82
collagen fibres 102
comfrey oil 19, 35, 54, 89, 105
compresses 49, 74, 82, 88, 89
congestion 25, 27, 31, 48, 80
conjunctivitis 31
"connective tissue massage" 112
constipation 21, 27, 28, 29, 30, 31, 35, 82, 88, 92, 103, 107
continuous circle strokes 67
contraceptive pill 22
convalescence 21, 22, 29, 33, 94–5
couches, massage 186
coughs 20, 21, 23, 24, 25, 26, 27, 28, 31, 32, 33, 90, 106
cramp 22, 25, 26
  abdomen 31, 83, 107
  calves 103, 181
  legs 177, 180–1
  muscles 23
creams, facial 55
cupping 69, 71, 113
Cupressus sempervirens 23, 106
cuts 20, 23, 24, 26, 27, 32, 33
Cymbopogon martini 30, 107
cypress oil 23, 35, 40, 47, 50, 52, 54, 56, 58, 80, 82, 84, 88, 97, 106, 179
cystitis 20, 21, 22, 23, 24, 26, 30, 32, 33, 35, 106

D

dandruff 21, 22, 32, 33, 35, 58, 106
De Chauliac, Guy 100
depression 20, 22, 24, 25, 26,

30, 31, 32, 33, 35, 106, 107
  post-natal depression 24
dermatitis 22, 24, 26, 29, 30, 31, 32, 51
detoxification 24, 26, 30, 61, 67, 72, 84, 85, 86–7, 103, 106, 177
diarrhoea 21, 23, 24, 25, 27, 29, 30, 32, 35, 82, 107
diet 9, 54, 58, 80, 84, 86
digestion 21, 25, 28, 29, 103, 106, 107
  massage therapies 82–3
  see also indigestion
dilution rates 15, 19, 34, 38, 47, 60, 92, 104–5
dreams, recalling 22

E

ears 22, 25, 27, 33
eczema 20, 24, 26, 31, 32, 35, 36, 51, 106
effleurage 66, 70, 91, 110, 112
elbows 53
  tennis elbow 181
elderly, massage 92–3
epilepsy 19, 32, 105
equipment for massage 63, 108–9, 186–7
  see also essential oils
essential oils 14–17, 20–33
  baths 50–1
  blending 19, 34, 36, 38, 43, 60, 105
  blends 40–3, 44
  carrier oils 36, 50, 104
  categories 39
  for fragrances 46–7
  inhaling 19, 44, 48, 80
  for massage 60, 104–7
  for problems 35
  sensual 185
  and states of mind 96–7
  storage 39